EXECUTIVE NUTRITION AND DIET

Other books available in this series

- COPING WITH EXECUTIVE STRESS
- EXECUTIVE FITNESS

EXECUTIVE NUTRITION AND DIET

Executive Health Examiners

Richard E. Winter, M.D.
Series Editor

McGraw-Hill Book Company

New York St. Louis San Francisco Auckland Bogotá Guatemala Hamburg
Johannesburg Lisbon London Madrid Mexico Montreal New Delhi Panama
Paris San Juan São Paulo Singapore Sydney Tokyo Toronto

The Author

Lawrence Galton is one of the most prolific medical/scientific writers in America today. As a medical columnist for FAMILY CIRCLE MAGAZINE and a contributing medical editor to PARADE MAGAZINE, Mr. Galton has contributed articles to over 50 national publications including READER'S DIGEST and THE NEW YORK TIMES. He has written or contributed to 19 books on health. He has received awards for his work from several associations, including the American Heart Association.

1234567890 DODO 898765432

ISBN 0-07-019861-6

This book was set in Zapf Book Light by Progressive Typographers; the editors were Robert P. McGraw and Maggie Schwarz; the production supervisor was Jeanne Skahan; the designer was Murray Fleminger. R. R. Donnelley & Sons Company was printer and binder.

See Acknowledgments on page 258.
Copyrights included on this page by reference.

Library of Congress Cataloging in Publication Data
Main entry under title:

Executive nutrition and diet.

  (Executive health series)
  Includes index.
  1. Executives—Nutrition. 2. Diet.
I. Executive Health Examiners (U.S.) II. Series.
TX361.E93E93   613.2'024658   82-15220
ISBN 0-07-019861-6   AACR2

Executive Health Examiners

Richard E. Winter, M.D.	*Chairman*
William S. Wanago, M.D.	*Senior Vice President of Medical Affairs*
John A. Rossa, M.D.	*Director, New York Executive Clinic*
Allyn Kidwell, M.D.	*Director, Morristown Executive Clinic*
John M. Hill, M.D.	*Director, Stamford Executive Clinic*
Gazanfer Alkaya, M.D.	*Director, New York Stock Exchange Clinic*
Charles Ulrich, M.D.	*Director, Ambulatory Health Service Clinic*
Neil Crane, M.D.	*Director, EHE Washington Bureau*
Julio Rivera, M.D.	*Director, Occupational Medical Service, NIH Clinic*
Barbara Wasserman, M.D.	*Director, Clinical Medicine, NIH Clinic*
John Foulke, M.D.	*Director, NASA Goddard Clinic*
Richard Ross, M.D.	*Director, Fairchild Republic Clinic*
Gitanjali Mukerjee, M.D.	*Director, Spofford Detention Center, Medical Service*
William McBride, M.D.	*Director, NASA Dryden Research Center, Medical Service*
Fred Block, M.D.	*Director, Chemical Bank Clinic*
Frank Marzullo, M.D.	*Director, Bank of New York Clinic*
Donna M. Hartl, M.D.	*Director, Johnson & Higgins Clinic*
Riska Platt, M.S., R.D.	*Director, Nutrition Programs*
Steven Tay, M.D.	*Associate Director, New York Executive Clinic*
Jack Goldman, M.D.	*Associate Director, New York Stock Exchange Clinic*
Socrates Fotiu, M.D.	*Associate Director, NASA Goddard Clinic*
Stanley Craig, M.D.	*Radiology*
Stanley Halprin, M.D.	*Cardiology*
Lawrence Koblenz, M.D.	*Gastroenterology*
Stephen Krasnica, M.D.	*Cardiology*
Mauro Mecca, M.D.	*Internal Medicine*
Bernard Nemoitin, M.D.	*Proctology*
Jasu Sanghvi, M.D.	*Gynecology*
Erasmo Sturla, M.D.	*Endocrinology*
Sidney Wanderman, M.D.	*Proctology*
Mel Weinstein, M.D.	*Internal Medicine*
Madeleine Steele	*Project Coordinator*

CONTENTS

PREFACE

Twenty-five years ago, in one of our preeminent medical research centers, there resided a group of very special laboratory animals. Challenged constantly, forced to make decisions and to act under pressure, they were the "executive monkeys." In one famous experiment, two monkeys were placed side-by-side in chairs equipped to give electric shocks. One of the monkeys—and only one—could prevent the shocks to both itself and its partner by pressing a lever. Under the psychological stress of being responsible for pressing the lever, this executive monkey developed duodenal ulcers.

The close correlation of behavior patterns in animals and humans has been thoroughly documented by scientific research. It has been shown that information obtained from animal research can be successfully applied to human research and experience. The study of animal behavior, for example, can result in a better understanding of the behavior of the individuals who go out each day to lead our governments, industries, and unions.

Few of us have ever watched chimpanzees in their natural habitat, the jungles of Africa. If we could observe these animals, we would see that they wander around, nibbling a few nuts here, a few berries there, eating continuously in small amounts. What they do *not* do is neglect eating for long periods and then pour raw alcohol onto the tender mucosal linings of their stomachs. They do *not* smoke several cigarettes, and thereby increase the outpouring of hydrochloric acid. They do *not* then consume large quantities of food, try to exist on insufficient sleep, and undergo rapid changes in environment. If they did, they would very likely suffer the same fate as a number of American executives under observation at a major research center who, possessing one or more of these habits, died before the study could be completed.

Medical science has accumulated an enormous amount of significant data from studies on animals and humans. As always, though, the important task is putting that knowledge to use in practical ways that can most benefit humankind. EXECUTIVE HEALTH EXAMINERS was founded more than twenty years ago for the primary purpose of making medical knowledge available to a particular group—executives. Over the years our medical staff has examined executives from every kind of business and profession and at every level. From this vast experience it has become apparent to us that these executives—men and women alike—are often *simultaneously* exposed to all the life-threatening habits that chimpanzees naturally avoid. And it is this circumstance that, in our opinion, makes executives unique. Other groups are, of course, subjected to some of the same threats to their health, but, in our experience, only in the executive lifestyle do these threats converge at the same time.

The conviction that executives are unique, that their lifestyles are different and therefore their health needs special, led us to prepare a series of books specifically for executives. In these volumes we combine solid medical fact with our years of professional experience to provide practical, proven approaches to solving health problems. Each volume deals with an area of health where executives are especially vulnerable. COPING WITH EXECUTIVE STRESS provides the most current medical information on stress and its effect on both the mind and body to show executives how to recognize and cope with stress in executive life. EXECUTIVE NUTRITION AND DIET is a commonsense program for nutrition and diet that has been highly successful for thousands of executives. All the special problems of executive lifestyle are dealt with in this basic, balanced discussion of sound nutritional habits and healthy diet. EXECUTIVE FITNESS is a flexible, workable exercise program designed for busy executives. Within a basic format, it offers a wide variety of exercise options, all of which are certain to result in increased stamina and productivity.

There is no question that the demands of executive life make good health maintenance difficult. Having guided hundreds of thousands of executives to positive and lasting changes in their lifestyle, however, we know that the habits of eating properly, exercising regularly and coping with stress can be successfully acquired. The volumes in this series offer sound information gained from long and specific experience with executives. We view these books as a kind of survival kit for executives. It is our hope that they will enable every executive to enjoy a longer, healthier, more productive and satisfying life.

Richard E. Winter, M.D.
Chairman

INTRODUCTION

Every executive knows it: What we put into the gut each day does more than stoke the body's furnace.

Today executives, as well as the general public, are becoming increasingly aware of the impact that nutrition has, both directly and indirectly, on health and disease—on heart disease, stroke, high blood pressure, diabetes, cancer, etc., as well as on vigor and longevity.

But confusion abounds. Almost weekly, new self-proclaimed diet prophets clamor for our attention. Food fads come and go. We hear endlessly about the pros and cons of vitamins and substances passed off as vitamins, of minerals, of fibers, and of food additives. The media are full of advice, much of it conflicting, about what to eat and what not to eat.

At Executive Health Examiners, many of our clients have expressed the need for reliable guidance not just to cut through the general confusion, but to help them deal with the special nutritional problems arising from the executive lifestyle and executive activities.

It was to address those problems that several years ago we set up a special department for nutritional counseling to supplement the work of our examining physicians.

This book stems from that counseling and the positive results experienced by many of our executive clients. We have tried to make it concise, direct, and practical.

* *What exactly are the lifestyle factors that impinge on executives and their diets? This is the concern of Chapter 1.*

* *Without an understanding of the three basic carriers of nutrition — proteins, fats, and carbohydrates—and the myths surrounding them, it is virtually impossible to avoid confusion.*

1

* *To determine whether or not you have a weight-control problem, read chapter 3. It examines the pitfalls of widely publicized diets, and then shows you how to proceed sensibly and soundly to get to your desired weight in the face of business lunches, travel, and entertainment.*

* *Chapter 4 clarifies the role of nutrition in heart and blood vessel disease and discusses what dietary measures can be preventive.*

* *Chapter 5 maps a path through the vitamin, mineral, and food fad maze.*

* *Chapter 6 provides pertinent, practical, useful information on when and how alcohol can be helpful; when and how an excess of caffeine in its many forms may be harmful; what dietary fiber is clearly able to do and what it may be able to do; and, not least of all, the relationship between nutrition and cancer.*

* *Finally, Chapter 7 is a succinct summation of the principles of ideal diet and includes useful guidelines for shopping, food preparation, and restaurant eating.*

1

[Mon]day

Tuesday 31

Wednesday 1

Thursday 2

Your mental health is ...
outside of this office

Monday:

8:30 JIM HENRY + PETE BAILEY

IRENE LASKEY

LAWYERS FOR R.W.I.

Lunch 12:30
R.P. + S.H. FROM DATA RESEARCH

[PER]SONNEL COMMITTEE

'83 BUD.

Tuesday 31:

STAFF - '83 BUDGET

Lunch OPERATIONS MANAGEMENT LUNCH

3:30 BOB HERBERT - MENLO INDUSTRIES

TOM WATSON

Eve ASSOCIATED MANUFACTURERS RECEPTION 6-8:30 COLONY CLUB

Wednesday 1:

7:30 BREAKFAST Ron Smith - WASH. OFF. ARLINGTON HOUSE

GOVERNMENT AFFAIRS COMMITTEE

Lunch SHUTTLE TO WASH. D.C.

JEFF HUGHES - F.T.C.

BEN RODGERS AT HOTEL

Eve RECEPTION FOR CONGRESSMAN WALKER HILTON - 6:30
BILL BENNETT - DINNER

Thursday 2:

BREAKFAST - SENATOR SCHMIDT + STAFF 8:

8:30 RALPH SIMMONS COMMERCE DEPT.

11:30

Lunch WASHINGTON STAFF 12:15 LUNCH AT JASON'S
Lunch 12:30 DELE[GATES]

JOHN ANDREWS - DEPT. OF JUSTICE
SYST[

SHUTTLE TO N.Y.
5:15 TONY

Eve PARENTS COMMITTEE RIVER COUNTRY DAY 8:00

NUTRITION AND THE EXECUTIVE LIFESTYLE

T.R.P. is a 53-year-old senior vice president in a large Manhattan-based corporation. At least 25 percent of his time is spent in travel, much of it around the United States and some of it abroad. When in town, he schedules three and four business luncheons each week. Of late, he has been having breakfast now and then with a client to get an early start on a productive day.

During the past 6 years, he has gained 45 unneeded pounds, his cholesterol level has risen sharply, and his blood pressure has increased to a level far higher than it should be.

Is T.R.P.'s executive lifestyle contributing significantly to his obesity and the potentially dangerous upsurge in his blood fats and blood pressure? He thinks it is and is concerned.

His is a concern that is shared by many other executives.

There are, of course, other elements making up the picture. Certainly, the nutrition of executives, like that of Americans in all walks of life, is influenced by social and cultural factors that have resulted in a national diet linked to major health problems—among them, obesity, heart and blood vessel diseases, stroke, high blood pressure, diabetes, cir-

BUT IN ALL CASES IT IS PRESENT

"The killer diseases of today are more insidious than the bacterial diseases that were serious causes of mortality and morbidity in the past, and they usually have a complex, noninfectious etiology.

"Atherosclerotic heart disease, hypertension, cancer, diabetes, and related diseases account for most postchildhood deaths in the United States. While causes of these diseases are quite different, they all have at least one thing in common—a nutritional component.

"In some cases the nature of that component is clear, in others obscure; in some cases simple, in others complicated, but in all cases it is present."

Myron Winick, M.D., Director,
Institute of Human Nutrition,
New York City

rhosis of the liver, and some cancers. In recent years this has led to growing general concern.

In common with much of the rest of the population, many executives are understandably confused about diet. One after another, new pied pipers appear with "miracle" diets—reducing diets, invigorating diets, long-life diets— some of which are bizarre, even dangerous.

Add, too, often-conflicting advice on what to eat and what not to eat from scientists, food producers, and, increasingly of late, government agencies.

"If you listen to everything you hear," lament executives as well as others, "you might as well throw up your hands and stop living or maybe become a vegetarian."

And beyond being exposed to the same influences and information shared by others, executives have particular patterns of work and living that all too easily can add to their nutritional problems.

How America Eats

Not long ago, in a series of articles on current eating patterns, a *New York Times* reporter wrote that although millions of Americans were supposed to have become concerned in recent years with good nutrition, there was no clear evidence "that even those people who say they are interested in improved nutrition have altered their eating

Executives have particular patterns of work and living that can add to their nutritional problems.

habits." According to D. Mark Hegsted, M.D., of the Human Nutrition Center of the U.S. Department of Agriculture, who was quoted in the *Times* article, "Americans now seem to be as fat as ever."

Writing in the *National Food Review*, two Agriculture Department scientists, Betty B. Peterkin and Ruth M. Marston, reported that Americans are managing to ignore all warnings that they are eating too much. "The caloric and most nutrient levels of the U.S. diet are the same as or higher than last year and ten years ago."

The Record

Here are a few figures worthy of inclusion in the *Guinness Book of World Records*:

* *American sugar consumption, now at its highest rate ever, averages 850 calories per person per day. Added at the table? Some, yes. But 82 percent of it goes into processed foods. Nor is it a matter of concern only in candies, ice cream, and baked desserts; sugar is an important ingredient in soups, sauces, cold breakfast cereals, vegetable juices, crackers, breads, and even salad dressings.*

* *Salt intake is excessively high; some estimates put it at an average of 15 grams (half an ounce) a day, far beyond any actual body requirement. Plenty is added at the table; plenty more is found in processed foods.*

* *Fat consumption, also at record levels, averages 52.6 pounds per person per year.*

* *Whereas the American per capita consumption of fresh fruits once averaged 134.7 pounds, this figure has recently hit a low of 83.2 pounds.*

* *Vegetable consumption has increased, but the bulk of vegetables being consumed are processed vegetables, the consumption of which has shot up from 14.5 pounds per person in 1910 to 62.5 pounds recently.*

* *Look what has happened to potato consumption: Even as late as 1950, almost all potatoes (94 percent) grown in the United States were eaten fresh; now most (60 percent) are processed, largely as frozen french fries, which from the tonnage standpoint have become the country's most-consumed vegetable.*

Goals and Guidelines

In 1977, concerned about a national diet rich in meats, dairy products, and processed foods laden with fats, cholesterol, sugar, salt, and calories, the U.S. Senate Select Committee on Nutrition and Human Health issued its "Dietary Goals" report.

The report advised Americans to cut down on fatty meats and dairy products, eggs, salty foods and snacks, and nutritionally deficient sweets and alcohol.

On the positive side, it advised eating more lean meats, fish and poultry, fruits, vegetables, whole grains, and other foods rich in complex carbohydrates, fiber, vitamins, and minerals and low in fat and refined sugars.

A controversial report! It had many in the food and dairy industries and even some independent scientists up in arms, arguing that such broad recommendations for dietary change on a vast national scale had to be considered premature and that enough clear evidence to provide justification was still lacking.

Yet, almost 3 years later, in what has been termed a "historic joint enterprise," two federal departments—the Department of Agriculture and the Department of Health, Education and Welfare (since renamed the Department of Health and Human Services)—joined forces to issue a "Dietary Guidelines for Americans" report.

Largely reinforcing the earlier report, the "Guidelines" urged: "Eat a variety of foods; maintain ideal weight; avoid too much fat, saturated fat and cholesterol; eat foods with adequate starch and fiber; avoid too much sugar; avoid too much sodium (salt); if you drink alcohol, do so in moderation."

In his first major speech, Secretary of Health and Human Services Richard S. Schweiker said: "By₃ taking five simple steps, by not smoking, by using alcohol in moderation, and by eating a proper diet and getting the proper amount of exercise and sleep, a 45-year-old man can expect to live 10 or 11 years longer than a person who does not make these choices."

The Argument

Proponents of dietary change relate the high incidence of heart and blood vessel diseases among Americans to the surge in consumption of animal foods, which are rich in cholesterol and fats, and which now account for 70 percent of the protein eaten by Americans, as compared with less than half that (30 percent) at the turn of the century.

These proponents argue that because of the relative decrease in consumption of whole grains as well as fresh fruits and vegetables, our diet is lacking in natural dietary fiber— and fiber, according to experimental evidence, can be helpful in combating obesity, diabetes, high blood pressure, and cancer of the colon.

They add that our heavy intake of sugar contributes little but needless calories and that our huge consumption of salt promotes hypertension.

To be sure, more definitive proof of the benefits of dietary modification would be welcome. In some studies dietary change appears to have reduced disease risk, but much of the evidence favoring change is based on epidemiologic (population) studies—studies indicating that around the world the more typically American the diet, the higher the

The more typically American the diet, the higher the death rate from atherosclerotic heart disease, high blood pressure, diabetes, and cancer of the colon.

death rate from such diseases as atherosclerotic heart disease, high blood pressure, diabetes, and cancer of the colon.

So, they argue that even short of the definitive proof that would be desirable, dietary change makes sense. It is hardly likely to be harmful.

Executive Eating (and Drinking) Patterns

While Americans in general have nutritional problems, those problems are aggravated for executives.

Consider the problem of R.S., a 54-year-old controller with an occupational hazard.

The company where R.S. works owns three gourmet restaurants in the New York metropolitan area that are notorious for their huge portions of prime-cut beef and other rich foods. One of the "better" fringe benefits is free food whenever an employee wants it.

As a result, R.S. had watched his weight increase by 2 pounds each year for the last 25 years. He knew he was at least 50 pounds over his ideal weight, but when his physician at Executive Health Examiners discovered an elevated fasting blood sugar, or glucose, level of 160 milligrams per deciliter of blood serum, he became frightened because diabetes runs in his family. The physician referred him to the nutritionist to discuss a weight-loss program, the primary treatment for adult-onset diabetes.

At Executive Health Examiners the nutritionist worked with R.S. on modifying his diet to include smaller portions of food at mealtimes. Gradually he was able to eliminate

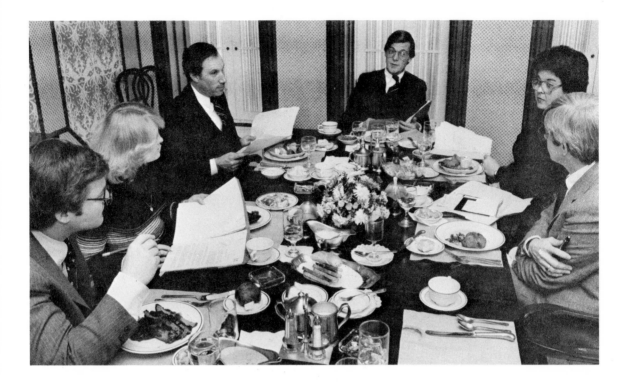

snacks and most of the desserts constantly available. He cooperated fully at home by cooking the foods suggested by the nutritionist. Within 9 months, R.S. lost 38 pounds and his blood glucose fell into the normal range (60 to 120 milligrams per deciliter of blood serum). He continues to work on losing that final 12 pounds but is gratified that he has maintained a 38-pound weight loss and normal fasting blood glucose.

You can do as well even if you eat as many restaurant meals as R.S.

The Business Lunch and Other Restaurant Meals

When a study of a large group of executives in one corporation was made by a senior nutritionist at the Massachusetts Institute of Technology, the biggest nutritional problem proved to be overabundance—of calories, fat, and protein.

The prime mistake of the executives was the consumption of excessively large portions of food—as much, for example, as 12 to 16 ounces of meat per meal, which is far beyond a normal serving of only about 4 ounces of boneless, cooked meat.

Overgenerous portions are to be found in many restaurants. Nor is it an easy matter for anyone brought up from childhood to "clean his or her plate" to do the opposite and reject excess.

Moreover, to many, it seems that when entertaining or being entertained it is inappropriate to appear "picky." Business meals often provide a rationale for eating what one should not because to do otherwise would be to "insult" one's host or guest.

There is also the element of time. Sitting over a meal for an extended period while business is discussed can invite more food consumption, even the ordering of an extra course.

Restaurant meals, furthermore, are often rich. Not only are desserts calorie- and fat-laden but also gravies, sauces, and salad dressings are. Even potatoes and other fresh vegetables may be prepared with fat.

Theoretically, broiled dishes should have a minimum of fat, but for restaurants, labor costs are greater than food costs and, whenever possible, methods of cooking are chosen on the basis of how expeditious they are. So it is often easier to broil something using a whole stick of butter than just a dab. With little butter, great care is needed if foods are not to dry out, stick, and become messy to clean up. It may help, when ordering, to specify that broiling be done without butter, in wine or lemon juice.

The Executive Dining Room

This is not necessarily a nutritional bargain. Executive dining rooms can have the same faults as many restaurants—portions that are too large and foods that are too rich.

And there may be an extra trap for the unwary. In some executive dining rooms, large round tables are set for many diners and the custom is to wait until a table fills before service is begun. Meanwhile, temptingly placed in the middle of the table are many dishes of cheese, crackers, pâté, and varied hors d'oeuvres. Much munching can go on before the table fills.

And Maybe—Now and Then—a Fast Food Lunch

Millions of such lunches, of course, are eaten every day across the country. On occasion, when he or she does not have a business lunch scheduled and is pressed for time, even an executive may duck into a fast-food emporium for a "hamburger and . . ." or may have such a lunch sent in to be eaten in the office.

Again, this is no bargain if you are watching your weight or your blood level of cholesterol and triglycerides.

Take the "quarter-pounder" hamburger. According to a recent U.S. Department of Agriculture sampling, you can count on getting 420 calories, 45 percent of which will come

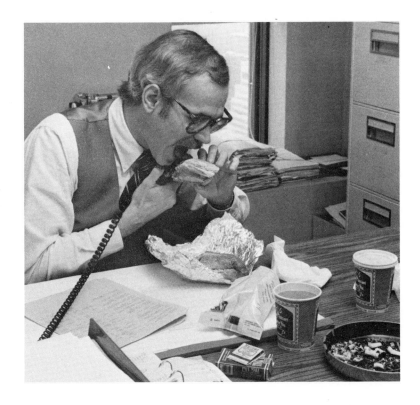

from fat, the vast proportion of it saturated fat. You will get a nice serving of cholesterol as well—77 milligrams worth.

Or take a quarter-pounder with cheese: the calories, 559; the proportion from fat, 49 percent; the milligrams of cholesterol, 110.

French fries to go with your burger? Figure on about 250 calories or even a bit more, with as much as 49 percent of them coming from fat—plus 12 milligrams of cholesterol. Potatoes have no cholesterol themselves and extremely small amounts of fats; the content of fats and cholesterol in french fries reflects the use of fat in the deep fryers.

Oh, yes, you may have condiments added to your burger. The calories vary, but they can range as high as 105 extra for one chain's special sauce and 159 extra for the mayonnaise usually added by another chain.

Alcohol

When he was asked whether alcohol makes much of a difference in the executive diet, Fredrick J. Stare, M.D., of the Harvard University Department of Nutrition, observed that next to meat, alcohol is the second major source of calories for the typical businessman.

"And," he went on, "you don't have to be a drunkard to get most of your calories from alcohol. Yesterday I had lunch with some board members in New York, and we went to a luncheon club. Practically every person I saw there had two drinks at lunch, big drinks, and there's a good 300 Calories.

"You get home and you have another good drink, a nice strong martini, say, and that's another 150. Now we're up to 450.

"Then, if you have wine with dinner, you're going to get another 100 Calories, and you're up to 550. In the evening, people often have another drink while they're looking over the papers, another 150 Calories, and maybe another one as a nightcap. So there's 800 or 900 Calories—which is a third of my daily caloric requirement—from alcohol."

Dr. Stare made those comments some years ago. From

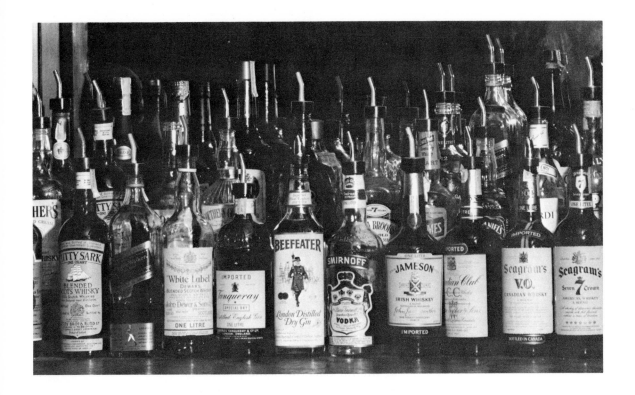

our observations at Executive Health Examiners, we think there has been some moderation since then in drinking by executives. Still, in many cases, alcohol contributes a significant number of calories—and no nutrients. The consumption of alcohol can be a particular problem for executives who do extensive traveling.

Travel

Among executives, travel is commonly very much part of the job. It is not unusual for them to spend as much as 25 percent or more of their time away from home.

Certainly, it is not impossible to eat well and moderately and to control one's weight while traveling, but it can be more difficult.

A SPECIAL NOTE ABOUT AIR TRAVEL

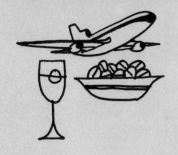

Particularly during long flights, air travel can present a special problem: *dehydration*.

As much as 2 pounds of water can be lost by evaporation through the skin during even a $3\frac{1}{2}$-hour flight in a commercial jet. This results from the rapid circulation of very dry air in the ventilating system.

Dehydration (fluid loss with insufficient replenishment) can, if allowed to progress, become severe enough to produce one or more symptoms such as flushing, dry skin and mucous membranes, cracked lips, decreased urination, lethargy, fatigue, low blood pressure, and muscle cramps.

But, far short of that, it can make for under-par feelings and can contribute to jet lag. One cannot depend on thirst to signal the need for adequate water consumption in this situation.

The emphasis should be on *water* consumption. It is not wise to depend on alcoholic beverages, since these, in fact, can contribute to further fluid loss. So can coffee, tea, and many soda beverages which contain enough caffeine to act as diuretics, increasing fluid excretion.

Insipid as airplane water may taste, drink it, or ask for bottled water or club soda.

From article by A. H. Hayes, *New York Times*, June 19, 1981.

When people travel, they often have a pronounced tendency to eat differently than they do at home.

Many of those who rarely have more for breakfast than juice, cereal, and coffee find themselves indulging in multi-course breakfasts. Dinners taken in restaurants are often more lavish than those eaten at home.

Some individuals may feel expansive about eating because it goes on the expense account; for others, indulging themselves by eating large meals of rich food may seem to offer some compensation, however little, for being away from home.

It is not impossible to eat well and moderately and to control one's weight while traveling, but it can be difficult.

The Woman Executive

Not only do women executives have problems similar to those of men (business lunches, frequent traveling), they may have some additional ones as well.

Women executives have even more reason for concern about their weight than do men. Generally, women have less lean body mass and lower metabolic rates, and it is easier for them to develop weight-control problems.

Women have more concerns, too, about meeting nutritional needs. They have greater susceptibility to anemia during the child-bearing years, because of inadequate iron intake to compensate for the loss in menstruation. Later, they are more susceptible to osteoporosis, or bone thinning and bone fractures.

For some, premenstrual tension may be a problem. The symptoms, such as irritability and fluid accumulation during the week or 10 days prior to menstruation, often can be relieved, and in some cases even completely eliminated, by reducing salt intake, but this can be difficult for women who must frequently eat in restaurants and corporate dining rooms or take all their meals out while traveling.

The Attack Starts Here

Is it possible for executives, given the realities of their work and lifestyles, to improve their nutritional habits and to attain better general health, including weight loss, lowered blood pressure, and reduced blood cholesterol and fat levels, if called for?

We can answer yes, on the basis of our experience with many thousands of executives.

Not by any means do all executives have nutritionally related problems. Many eat well and enjoy excellent health. They have developed simple, practical techniques to assure this, techniques which fit in well with their work and have become entirely comfortable parts of their lives. They are techniques worth noting—and we will be noting them.

Others have had problems—some relatively mild, some quite serious, even alarming.

WHAT ABOUT WATER?

About 60 percent of total body weight is water, and all the chemical reactions in your body that convert food to energy and body tissue require its presence. The body retains the amount of water you need at any given time, and when you are running low, you feel thirsty. When you have taken in more than you need, the kidney receives a hormonal message to rid your body of the excess as urine.

Though some elderly or ill people can develop thirst-control abnormalities, most people go a life-time without any water metabolism problems.

Executive Health Examiners recommends that, unless advised aganst it by a doctor, adults drink between 6 and 8 cups of liquids daily. Coffee, tea, cola beverages, and alcohol do not count as satisfying this requirement.

Not only do women executives have problems similar to those of men—they have additional ones as well.

Here is an extreme case, one of the potentially most serious:

P.W. was a man in his midforties when he was first examined at Executive Health Examiners. Markedly obese, he exceeded his ideal weight by 100 pounds. His cholesterol level was 274 milligrams per deciliter of blood serum, which is in the above-normal range, and his blood serum level of triglycerides (a fatty component in the blood) was markedly elevated at 460 milligrams per deciliter.

His blood pressure was of even more concern: 200/130. A marked elevation—and apparently so long sustained that the examination showed deterioration of the blood vessels in his eyes as a consequence. His legs, too, were puffed up—edematous—suggesting an effect on his heart and circulation from the hypertension.

Still another indication of his poor condition was a resting pulse rate of 100 beats per minute, above the normal range of 60 to 80 beats per minute. He was in miserable condition.

We were concerned, but he professed not to be. Our chief medical officer spent an hour with him trying to make him concerned. "Forget it," he said. "I feel fine."

A year later he was back with no improvement whatever, weighing 10 more pounds, and with the same response to our medical concern but with this bit of amplification: "Look, the only reason I go through this yearly examination business is because my company insists."

The year before, we had sent P.W. a straightforward written report noting the facts about his health and urging action. He got a written message now that pulled no punches. It said in part:

You are found to be in poor health. You suffer from a marked overweight problem; you also have significant hypertension. Your laboratory abnormality—triglyceride elevation—is a direct result of your weight and will predispose you to the development of early coronary disease and a possible premature heart attack.

It is our responsibility to warn you that the present state of your health is a semiemergency situation and not something to consider lightly. If immediate efforts are not made to improve or correct your problems, you may possibly suffer severe consequences to your health.

People can do remarkable things when properly motivated. And this man was motivated now. As he confessed later, "That report letter seemed to me like a death warrant —in black and white. I had never had it put to me that way before."

P.W. lost 110 pounds in little more than a year. Once he had lost it, he went out and spent $2000 on a new wardrobe as an incentive to maintain the lower weight. His blood pressure, thanks to the weight loss, dropped to 120/90 (normal) from the earlier 200/130 elevation; his cholesterol level went down from 274 to 200 milligrams per deciliter; and his triglyceride level had plummeted from 460 to a beautiful 67 milligrams per deciliter.

That was 4 years ago.

And today? His weight is right where he got it to 4 years ago, 174 pounds; his blood pressure remains normal; his triglycerides are still at the low level of 67 milligrams per deciliter; and his cholesterol is down a bit further to 194 milligrams per deciliter.

"I have never felt better in my life," he says, which is easy enough to understand.

Given motivation, even extreme changes—and certainly the far lesser ones usually needed—can be achieved, provided that the confusion surrounding nutrition is cut through to get to the relatively simple heart of the matter.

We will start with the cutting through in the next chapter.

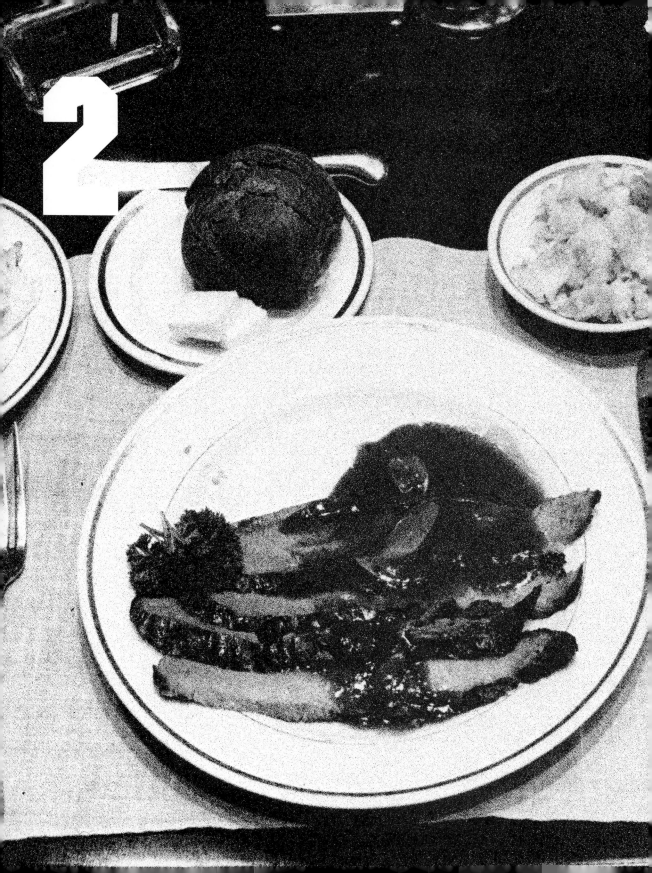

Carbos   55%
fats   30
proteins   15
          ‾‾‾‾
          100

The three basic carriers of nutrients

THE THREE BASICS: PROTEINS, FATS, AND CARBOHYDRATES

Of the many myths and misconceptions surrounding nutrition, these three are among the most common:

* *Because protein is the quintessential nutrient, there is no such thing as too much.*

* *As for fats, when it comes to good health, it's all just a matter of eating fewer saturated and more unsaturated fats.*

* *Carbohydrates (starchy foods) are our major miscreants: high in calories, not really needed, to be avoided as much as possible.*

All three are total nonsense! Proteins, fats, and carbohydrates are the vital dietary components, the calorie carriers, the three central substances of nutrition. Not only do all three have fundamental roles to play in the body's economy, so do their interactions.

Proteins

The myth: Second only to water, protein is the most important nutrient.
The facts: Protein is important all right, but the body's

21

need for it is quite limited. Many Americans, thinking there can't be too much of a good thing, consume far more than they need. The excess, however, is converted into sugar and fat, which are stored by the body if they are not immediately needed for energy.

Also, most high-protein foods include more fat besides the fat from the conversion of excess protein. It is stored, too, if it is not immediately needed.

Thus, besides adding extra calories to the diet, eating excess protein results in the addition of extra fat in more than one way.

What Proteins Do

The heart, liver, kidneys, muscles, brain tissue, hair, and nails all consist mainly of protein. No cell in the body can survive without an adequate protein supply. The very wall of a cell is protein, and protein makes up 20 percent of total cell mass.

Proteins build and maintain all body tissues by contributing the essential amino acids of which they are made. The amino acids are used to make enzymes (which further the body's chemical reactions), hormones, and body fluids. They help form antibodies to combat disease and blood hemoglobin to carry oxygen to tissues. They also contribute to the regulation of digestion and other body functions.

What Proteins Are

The most complex of natural compounds, proteins are built of small constituent units called amino acids (often referred to as the "building blocks" of protein) which contain nitrogen, carbon, and other elements.

What determines the nature of any particular kind of protein is the number and arrangement of those building blocks. For example, the protein albumin (a major constituent of albumen, or egg whites, and other animal-product foods) consists of 418 amino acids strung together in a particular way to form each albumin molecule.

It is not the complexity of proteins, however, which counts in the diet, but rather their amino acid constituents.

As you digest proteins, they are quickly broken down into their amino acid constituents, from which the body then builds the particular types of proteins that it requires— structural proteins and connective tissue proteins—as well as hormones, antibodies, enzymes, and other body substances. In fact, according to current estimates, in this building process the body produces as many as 50,000 different types of proteins.

More than twenty different amino acids are to be found in proteins. The body can synthesize many from sources of nitrogen and from the intermediate compounds that are formed as carbohydrates are broken down.

But there are some amino acids which the body is unable to synthesize and which are therefore dietary essentials. These "essential" amino acids include lysine, valine, isoleucine, leucine, threonine, tryptophan, methionine, phenylalanine, and histidine. Two other amino acids can be

THE PROTEIN CONTENT OF SOME FOODS

Food	Serving	Protein, g
Bread, wheat	1 slice	2–3
Cereals	½ cup	1–3
Cheese, cheddar	1 oz	7
Cheese, cottage	2 oz	10
Dried beans or peas	½ cup cooked	7–8
Egg	1 medium	6
Fish	3 oz	15–25
Fruits	½ cup	1–2
Meat	3 oz	15–25
Milk, whole	1 cup	9
Pasta	½ cup	2
Peanut butter	2 tbsp	8
Poultry	3 oz	15–25
Rice	½ cup	2
Vegetables	½ cup	1–3

derived only from amino acids which are dietary essentials: tyrosine from phenylalanine and cystine from methionine.

Protein Sources

All flesh—from fish, fowl, cattle, and other mammals—is rich in proteins. Cow's milk has a high protein content—in fact, three times as much as human milk. Some cheeses have still more. Cereals contain about 5 to 10 percent protein by weight. Fruits contain little protein—about 1 percent by weight. Vegetables, particularly peas and beans, have a greater proportion than fruit.

Foods that contain large amounts of the essential amino acids are known as *complete protein sources.* These include such animal-product foods as meat, eggs, and milk.

Vegetable proteins are incomplete; that is, no single vegetable contains all of the essential amino acids, but all of the amino acids can be obtained from a mix of vegetables. For example, Mexicans have a complete protein intake when they eat tortillas (corn bread), which are low in lysine, along with beans, which are rich in lysine and low in methionine.

Other complete protein sources include the following combinations of foods: peanut butter and whole wheat

RECOMMENDED DAILY DIETARY ALLOWANCES FOR PROTEIN AND ENERGY*

| | Age, years | Weight | | Energy, Cal | Protein, g | Protein, % of total calories |
		kg	lb			
Males	19–22	70	154	2900	56	7.7
	23–50	70	154	2700	56	8.3
	51+	70	154	2400	56	9.3
Females	19–22	55	120	2100	44	8.4
	23–50	55	120	2000	44	8.8
	51+	55	120	1800	44	9.8

* During pregnancy, the need for calories is increased by 300 grams and for protein by 30 grams; during lactation, caloric needs are increased by 500 grams and protein needs by 20 grams.

bread, rice and beans, nuts and beans, macaroni and cheese, and cereal and milk.

Protein Requirements

Although proteins are vital, body requirements for them are relatively low. Needs vary with age and size. The Food and Nutrition Board of the National Research Council has developed recommended daily allowances (RDAs) for proteins. These represent the minimum amounts needed per day—plus an extra, or safety, allowance of about 50 percent—to meet the needs at different ages of virtually all healthy people. (Protein requirements may be significantly increased during episodes of severe stress, infection, or injury.)

As you see from the table "Recommended Daily Dietary Allowances for Protein and Energy," the RDA for protein for a 70-kilogram (154-pound) man is 56 grams (about 2 ounces) a day, which is less than 10 percent of the RDA for calories.

Too Much Protein?

Most Americans get plenty of protein. In the United States, approximately 15 to 17 percent of total caloric intake is in the form of protein—some 90 to 100 grams a day.

According to a recent report by John D. Palombo and George L. Blackburn, M.D., of Harvard Medical School, "Ninety-seven percent of healthy Americans consume much more protein than is required; the amount of extra dietary protein consumed may approach 40 to 50 grams per day."

It is also a fact that the kind of protein consumed has

Ninety-seven percent of healthy Americans consume much more protein than is required.

changed since the turn of the century. More than two-thirds of dietary protein now comes from animal sources, as contrasted with one-half in 1900, when grain consumption was greater.

Extra protein contributes to obesity. A gram of protein has an energy value of about 4 calories, which is exactly the same as the energy value for a gram of carbohydrate. Moreover, foods don't contain protein alone:

* *In terms of calories, T-bone steak is about 20 percent protein and 75 percent fat.*

* *Cheddar cheese is 25 percent protein and 75 percent fat.*

* *Filet of sole, on the other hand, is only 10 percent fat.*

* *Chicken has more protein ounce for ounce than steak, while steak has $2\frac{1}{2}$ times more calories and twice as much fat.*

* *In other foods high in protein, carbohydrates provide most of the calories. For example, skim milk is 40 percent protein and 60 percent carbohydrate; kidney beans, 25 percent protein and 70 percent carbohydrate; whole wheat bread, 16 percent protein and 80 percent carbohydrate.*

Nutritionists generally recommend that proteins constitute between 10 and 15 percent of the daily caloric intake; the Senate Select Committee put the desired figure at 12 percent; and, as already noted, the Food and Nutrition Board's RDAs for protein are under 10 percent.

Reducing protein intake will, at the same time, almost certainly reduce the intake of fat, which so often goes along

Chicken has more protein ounce for ounce, than steak, while steak has $2\frac{1}{2}$ times more calories and twice as much fat.

LOW-FAT PROTEIN FOODS

Food	Fat, g
Skimmed milk, 9 oz	0.1
Uncreamed cottage cheese, 2 oz	0.17
Cooked shrimp, 1½ oz	0.5
Cooked rice and beans, 1½ cups	0.7
Chicken (no skin), 1½ oz	1.5
Pink salmon (canned), 1¾ oz	3.0
Haddock, 1¾ oz	3.3
Veal (trimmed), 1½ oz	4.5
Low-fat yogurt, 10 oz	5.0
Hamburger (lean), 1½ oz	5.0
Hamburger (regular), 1½ oz	8.5
Eggs (large), 1½ oz	10.0
Ham, 1½ oz	10.0
American cheese, 1½ oz	13.0

SOURCE: *Nutrition and Health* 1(5): 4, 1979.

with protein. That should bring a significant reduction in total calories, since fat contains more than twice as many calories as does protein or carbohydrates: 9 calories per gram.

THIS MATTER OF CALORIES

Look *calorie* up in a dictionary and you will find it defined as the amount of heat required to raise the temperature of 1 gram of water 1 degree Celsius (centigrade). However, in most discussions of nutrition—and throughout this book—*calorie* is commonly used to denote the amount of heat required to raise the temperature of 1 *kilo*gram of water 1 degree Celsius; used in this sense, it is also sometimes called a *large calorie* and is equivalent to 1 kilocalorie of heat.

Dictionary definitions also explain that *calorie* is a unit of measure expressing the heat- or energy-producing value in food when the food is oxidized in the body. Thus, it is not a food element, but rather a measure of the energy that can be produced by food when it is digested.

Originally, calorie was a unit of heat used by physicists. With it they could compare, for example, the amount of heat produced by burning a pound of coal (3 million calories) with the amount produced by burning a cubic foot of gas (125,000 calories).

Determining caloric values in food is relatively simple—a matter of measuring the heat produced when a food is burned in a bomb calorimeter.

The equipment consists of three vessels. The first, or outermost vessel is made of heavy metal and is designed to resist internal pressure. The second, or middle, vessel is insulated with cork to resist heat loss; it is placed inside the first vessel. The third, or innermost, vessel is filled with water, and a "bomb" containing a weighed amount of foodstuff and oxygen is placed inside it. It is then placed inside the middle vessel. The foodstuff is ignited electrically, and the heat produced is measured by determining the rise in the temperature of the water surrounding the bomb and converting it to calories—1 (large) calorie for each degree Celsius rise in temperature of 1 kilogram (2.2 pounds) of water.

Carbohydrates and proteins yield 4 calories per gram, or 128 calories per ounce, and fats yield 9 calories per gram, or 288 calories per ounce.

Given these figures and knowing the carbohydrate-protein-fat composition of any food, it is a simple matter to calculate the caloric value of any given amount of that food.

For example, an egg contains, along with fluid, about 13 percent protein, 10 percent fat, and no carbohydrates; therefore, an egg weighing 50 grams would contain 6.5 grams of protein and 5 grams of fat and would yield a total of 71 calories—45 from fat and 26 from protein.

A lump of sugar weighing half an ounce (approximately 15 grams) contains only carbohydrate, so it provides 60 calories from 4 calories per gram carbohydrate yield.

Fats

The myth: Maintaining a good ratio between saturated and unsaturated fats is an "open sesame" to good health.

Contrary to common belief, people who engage in strenuous exercise do *not* need to increase protein intake.

"Vigorous sports do not increase the need for protein," says Jean Mayer, M.D. "One hundred years of experiments and measurements have failed to show any beneficial effect of high-protein diet. If anything, muscles hang on to their protein a little better if they are exercised. An amount of protein reasonable for a non-athlete is quite adequate for the athlete, too."

Not only is there no increase in protein requirements with exercise, the fact is that protein is never a source of immediate energy and the body has no way to store extra protein as protein.

Protein must be used immediately or it is broken down by the liver and excreted by the kidneys. If you take in protein beyond what your body can use, you may not only be denying yourself other important nutrients but you may force your liver and kidneys to work harder.

The facts: The ratio between saturated and unsaturated fats is significant, true, but equally important is the *total intake* of fats.

The American diet has a higher fat content than almost any other in the world. Although agreement is not universal, many scientists blame our high-fat diet for a number of our major health problems, including obesity, heart disease, and possibly cancer of the colon and the breast.

What Fats Do

Fats serve many important and diverse purposes. Among other things, they do the following:

*   *Carry essential fatty acids the body needs but cannot produce for itself.*

*   *Become the primary form of energy reserve once they are absorbed. They are highly efficient energy storers. Any given weight of stored, or depot, fat will yield about $2\frac{1}{4}$ times as much energy as an equivalent weight of protein or carbohydrate.*

* *Form essential constituents of cell membranes that regulate cellular intake and excretion of all nutrients.*

* *Act as an insulator to maintain body temperature by being stored as reserves, mostly in fat layers under the skin.*

* *Hold organs, such as the heart and the kidneys, in place and protect them.*

* *Transport and aid in the absorption of essential fat-soluble vitamins; A, D, E, and K.*

* *Spare protein from use by the body for purposes other than tissue biosynthesis.*

* *Improve the palatability of food and stimulate the flow of digestive juices.*

* *Contribute to the health of the skin.*

What Fats Are

Fat molecules are similar to carbohydrates in that they contain carbon, hydrogen, and oxygen, but there is less oxygen in fat molecules. Also, the structural arrangement of fat molecules is such that carbon atoms are mostly tied to hydrogen atoms in a long string, whereas in carbohydrate molecules, oxygen atoms are mostly tied to hydrogen atoms. Thus, without hydrogen-oxygen links, there is no water held in fat molecules.

In effect, they are "dry," or at least relatively water-free; hence, they burn better, and provide greater caloric energy —more than twice as much as carbohydrates (or proteins).

The American diet has a higher fat content than almost any other in the world.

Many scientists blame our high-fat diet for a number of our major health problems including obesity, heart disease, and possibly cancer of the colon and breast.

For example, an ounce of fat can supply 240 calories, compared to 110 calories supplied by an ounce of carbohydrate or protein.

The carbon, hydrogen, and oxygen atoms in fats combine to form glycerol (a form of alcohol) plus fatty acids, which can be classified as *saturated* or *unsaturated*.

The saturated fatty acids have molecules constructed with single bonds between the carbon and hydrogen atoms and they contain all the hydrogen they can hold; in other words, they are saturated with hydrogen.

Unsaturated fatty acids, on the other hand, have some

FATTY ACID CONTENT OF SOME FATS AND OILS

	Percentage of total fatty acids		
	Saturated	*Monounsaturated*	*Polyunsaturated*
Butterfat	65.5	30.6	3.9
Beef fat (tallow)	50.4	44.3	5.3
Chicken fat	34.0	47.5	18.5
Coconut oil	91.7	6.4	1.9
Corn oil	13.3	25.9	60.8
Lard (pork fat)	41.4	46.3	12.3
Olive oil	14.8	75.8	9.4
Palm oil	50.1	40.2	9.7
Peanut oil	20.0	48.4	31.6
Safflower oil	9.8	13.0	77.2
Soybean oil	15.7	24.1	60.2
Sunflower oil	11.1	29.1	59.8

double bonds. They can take on more hydrogen under certain conditions. Some contain one double bond and are known as *monounsaturated;* others contain two or more double bonds and are called *polyunsaturated.*

All the common unsaturated fatty acids are liquid at room temperature. If hydrogen is added to unsaturated fatty acids, they become saturated and are converted into solid fats. This process is called *hydrogenation.*

Research has indicated that unsaturated fats are less likely than saturated fats to be harmful to the body. It appears that the normal blood concentration of cholesterol is increased by saturated fats, which are found mainly in meat, butter, and lard. On the other hand, unsaturated fats, found in large amounts in such vegetable oils as corn and safflower oil, help reduce the amount of cholesterol in the blood.

Some investigators believe that eating foods rich in cholesterol itself, such as egg yolks and liver, kidney, and other organ meats, also increases blood cholesterol levels. Excessive blood cholesterol is believed to be a major factor in atherosclerosis, in which fatty deposits form in arteries, such as those feeding the heart muscle, impeding blood flow and leading to coronary heart disease and heart attack.

Sources of Fat

Dietary fats come from cooking fats and oils, butter, margarine, salad dressings and oils, meats, whole milk, cream, cheese, ice cream, nuts, chocolate, and avocados.

Fat Requirements

Although Americans have become increasingly fat-conscious, most of us consume far more fats than we realize—or need.

Unsaturated fats are less likely than saturated fats to be harmful to the body.

Fats such as the hard-fat strips on meats, the fats and oils used for cooking, and the oil in salad dressing are visible fats, but most of the fats in our diet are not obvious.

The marbling in meats is not always readily apparent, and such foods as cream and hard cheeses, deep-fried dishes, creamed soups, chocolate, and ice cream are all laden with fat.

Virtually all the calories in nuts (about 85 percent) are provided by fats. Seeds (among them sunflower seeds)? Avocados? Credit some 75 percent of their calories to fat content.

Tuna, salmon, and oil-packed sardines are high in fat. So, too, are frankfurters, bologna, and salami—not to mention gravies and sauces, cakes, pies, cookies, snack foods, whipped toppings, and coffee whiteners!

Look at the ingredients of a quiche, and you find cheese (some 75 percent of its calories come from fat), cream (almost all fat), and crust (almost 50 percent fat).

Rich desserts? You expect them to have plenty of sugar, but they may contain even more fat.

Examine the labels of processed foods in your pantry or refrigerator. When fat is at or near the top of the ingredient list, obviously the product is high in fat.

Given label information on the grams of fat in a serving, you can determine the percent of fat calories. Multiply the number of fat grams per serving by 9 (the number of calories per gram of fat), then divide the result by the number of calories listed per serving and multiply by 100.

In 1901, fat made up 32 percent of the American diet; currently, it constitutes 42 percent. The increase has resulted chiefly from greater use of vegetable oils. Thanks to them, we consume much more polyunsaturated fat than before but without cutting back significantly on saturated fat and hydrogenated oils.

Animal-fat intake has remained around 100 grams per person per day. The proportion of animal fat to vegetable fat in the total fat supply decreased from 5 to 1 in 1909 to 1.5 to 1 in 1974. Vegetable fat used in margarine, shortening, oil, and salad dressing has supplanted much of the fat previously supplied by dairy products, butter, and lard.

But total fat intake is still too high.

Guidelines developed for the general public by the American Heart Association and the Inter-Society Commission for Heart Disease Resources recommend that only 30 to 35 percent of calories be supplied as fat.

Dietary goals recommended by the U.S. Senate Select Committee on Nutrition and Human Needs include a 25 percent reduction in fat intake.

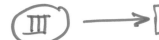

Carbohydrates

The myth: Foods containing lots of carbohydrates—both from starches and from sugars—are high in calories and low in nutritional values.

The facts: They are neither. On the contrary, carbohydrate-containing foods are effective carriers of many vital nutrients and are our major source of plant fiber, vitamin C, and the B vitamins—niacin, thiamin, and riboflavin—as well as of many important trace elements.

Ounce for ounce, carbohydrates are no more fattening than protein and have less than half the calories of fat.

Eat a 5-ounce potato without butter or sour cream, and you consume 110 calories. A 5-ounce steak, on the other hand, contains 500 calories because steak has more fat than protein. Yet weight watchers too often mistakenly leave potatoes on the plate and eat every last bite of steak.

What Carbohydrates Do

The major role of carbohydrates is to supply energy. In so doing, they spare protein so it can be used for its primary purpose of building and repairing body tissues. Carbohydrates also help the body utilize other nutrients, such as fiber, vitamins, and minerals.

The body's method of dealing with carbohydrates is to convert them to blood sugar, or *glucose*. Starches are converted into glucose by enzymes in the intestine; the body could not absorb them otherwise. Cane or beet sugar (sucrose) is converted into glucose plus fructose by the enzyme sucrase; the liver then changes the fructose into glucose. The enzyme lactase converts milk sugar into glucose plus galactose, and the liver then changes the galactose into glucose.

GLUCOSE

Energy from carbohydrates is quickly available and quickly used. Generally, within about a dozen hours the last

> In those who follow faddist low-carbohydrate diets, ketone bodies can accumulate in the blood, causing nausea, fatigue, and apathy.

of the carbohydrates from a meal have been burned up. Unless more energy from carbohydrates has become available in the meantime, fat stores are then ransacked for energy.

Supplying energy by burning fat is not highly efficient. In the process, ketone bodies (toxic breakdown products of the burning) are produced and have to be excreted by the kidneys. In those who follow faddist low-carbohydrate diets, ketone bodies can accumulate in the blood, causing nausea, fatigue, and apathy.

If for lack of adequate carbohydrates, the body also has to turn to proteins for energy, there can be more than one penalty. The amount of protein available for building and replacing tissues is reduced, and with the burning of protein, nitrogen is left over that must be excreted by the kidneys, which further adds to their burden.

What Carbohydrates Are

Carbohydrates, which include all sugars and starches, are made up of carbon, hydrogen, and oxygen. Just as in water, there are two hydrogen atoms for each atom of oxygen. Carbohydrates get their name because, in effect, they are hydrated (watered) carbons. They are best pictured as long chains of small building blocks. For example, starch, a large carbohydrate molecule, is a string of smaller, simpler sugar molecules.

There are many sugars: *Fructose*, the sweetest sugar (also known as *levulose* and *fruit sugar*), occurs in honey, ripe fruits, and many vegetables; *lactose* is a sugar in milk; *maltose* is a sugar from malt or digested starch; and *sucrose* is the table sugar in sugar cane and beets (from which comes table sugar), the sap from maple trees, and sorghum.

SUGARS

STARCHES

The starches, which are made up of complex sugars (polysaccharides rather than disaccharides such as sucrose), are not sweet like the simpler sugars. There are starches in tubers such as potatoes; in seeds such as peas, beans, peanuts, and almonds; and in roots such as carrots and beets. Our principal sources of starch, however, are ce-

CARBOHYDRATE CONTENT OF SOME FOODS

	Digestible carbohydrate, g
Bread, white or whole grain, 1 slice	13
Cereals:	
Bran flakes, 1 cup	28
Corn flakes, sugared, 1 cup	36
Oatmeal, 1 cup	23
Chocolate, 1 oz	14
Dried beans, cooked, $\frac{1}{2}$ cup	17–26
Dried peas, cooked, $\frac{1}{2}$ cup	17–26
Fruits:	
One fresh orange	16
Four dried prunes	18
Milk, 1 cup	12
Nuts, $\frac{1}{4}$ cup	4–10
Pasta, cooked, $\frac{1}{2}$ cup	16
One potato ($2\frac{1}{4}$-in diameter)	17
Rice, cooked, $\frac{1}{2}$ cup	25
Soft drinks, 8 oz	21–33
Sugar, 1 tbsp	11
Syrup (honey, molasses), 1 tbsp	13
Vegetables, cooked:	
Green beans, $\frac{1}{2}$ cup	4
Green peas, $\frac{1}{2}$ cup	10

real grains—wheat, rye, rice, barley, corn, millet, and oats—with which more than two-thirds of the world's croplands are planted.

Carbohydrate Requirements

Traditionally, carbohydrates have been the principal source of calories. Even now, for many in the world, 60 to 75 percent of food calories come from carbohydrates.

In the United States, however, carbohydrate consumption has fallen off markedly. At the turn of the century carbohydrates provided close to 50 percent of the calories in the diet; more recently the figure has fallen to 46 percent. The most marked decline has been in the consumption of nourishing complex carbohydrates, which has been partly offset by an increase in the consumption of "empty" calories in presweetened foods.

As a recent "white paper" of the American Dietetic Association points out, 1 pound of sugar was consumed in 1909 for every 10 pounds of fruit, vegetables, and cereal products, but "we now eat 1 pound of sugar for every 5 pounds of fruit, vegetables, and cereals. We are not eating the starchy vegetables and cereals that provide a balance between complex and simple carbohydrate, and also provide vitamins, minerals, and fiber."

The dietary goals recommended by the Senate Select Committee on Nutrition and Human Needs call for carbohydrates—especially the complex starches and naturally occurring sugars in fruits and vegetables—to make up 60 percent of our daily caloric intake.

FACTS TO CONSIDER ABOUT COMPLEX CARBOHYDRATES

- Unrefined or whole fruits, vegetables, and grains are important for supplying fiber, carbohydrate, vitamins, minerals, and calories.
- Enrichment of refined carbohydrates restores only a few of the vitamins and minerals lost in the refining process.
- The American diet has become very high in refined carbohydrate and, therefore, very low in dietary fiber.
- Low-fiber diets have been associated with constipation,

- diverticulitis, cancer of the colon, appendicitis, hemorrhoids, and hiatus hernia.
- Dietary fiber tends to hold water and produces stools that are bulkier, softer, and pass more quickly and easily through the intestines.
- A sudden, large increase in dietary fiber may cause uncomfortable flatulence, cramping, and distention. Add fiber *gradually* to your diet.
- Drink plenty of liquids, especially with more fiber in your diet. Liquids help to avoid gas, constipation, and intestinal blockage.
- The best way to increase dietary fiber is to increase unrefined, high-fiber foods such as whole grains, whole fruits, and vegetables.
- Whole grains spoil and turn rancid more quickly than refined grains. Store tightly sealed in a cool place.

Sugar—Sweet and Dangerous

Sugar was once affordable only for the rich—and even they couldn't get much of it. Apothecaries were the only sellers, and they measured it out by the ounce. In Elizabethan times, England consumed a grand total of only 88 tons of sugar a year.

Then, less than a century ago, Latin America began to cultivate sugar cane and a process was worked out in Europe for refining sugar beets. By 1850 annual world production had reached only 3.5 million tons, but by 1950 it was up to 35 million tons. Currently it is more than 70 million tons.

Per capita consumption of sugar per year in the United States, and in many other Western industrialized nations, now averages almost 140 pounds, more than 2 pounds per week.

Per capita consumption of sugar per year in the United States . . . averages almost 140 pounds, more than 2 pounds per week.

The consumption of sugar has long been of concern—at first, primarily in connection with tooth decay. As far back as the sixteenth century, it was remarked that Queen Elizabeth had a great fondness for sweetmeats made from sucrose extracted from cane, as witnessed by her black teeth. Since that time there have been numerous scientific studies linking sugar and tooth decay.

Many factors may enter into decay, but at the heart of the process is the activity of bacteria which produce acid that attacks the dentine. The bacteria have been shown to thrive on sweets, particularly sweets that stick to the teeth.

Sugar and Obesity

Sugar is certainly not the only contributor to obesity—no one particular food is—but a larger proportion of daily calories is provided by sugar than by anything else.

One of the best-known opponents of sugar is Britain's John Yudkin, M.D., biochemist and physician. Many people, Dr. Yudkin believes, could lose excess weight simply by giving up or severely restricting their intake of sugar. If, he points out, you take just 1 spoonful of sugar in each cup of coffee or tea and drink only 5 cups a day, you could lose more than 10 pounds a year by eliminating the sugar.

Moreover, Yudkin notes, sugar does more than contribute to obesity in and of itself:

> We have developed a liking for it that can increasingly be satisfied by a wide range of foods and drinks that many of us find almost irresistible. We take them more and more even though we don't need them. Some of the high amount of fat we eat comes [from] the use of sugar with fat in such foods as cakes, ice cream, and other sorts of confectionery. Sugar thus becomes a fat-carrier as well as providing calories itself.

Diabetes and Heart Disease

Aside from possibly contributing to diabetes and heart disease via obesity, does sugar do so directly? There have been some suggestive, but not definitive, studies.

Investigations in Israel found that the incidence of diabe-

DRINK BEVERAGES THAT CONTAIN LITTLE OR NO SUGAR

Many people drink a lot of cola and other soft drinks without realizing the amount of sugar and extra calories they contain. Consider the fact that each 12-ounce can of soda contains approximately 150 calories—all from sugar! (There are approximately 15 calories per level teaspoon of sugar.) In fact, drinking soda is probably worse than eating pure sugar because sodas often contain food coloring, caffeine, and other additives as well as empty calories. Consider some alternatives:

Have	Instead of	Sugar saved	Calories saved
Club soda with a twist of lemon or lime	Colas or other sweet sodas	10 tsp per 12 oz	150 per 12 oz
Fruit juices mixed half and half with club soda	Fruit drinks or pure fruit juice	3–4 tsp per 4 oz	45–60 per 4 oz
Unsweetened tea or coffee*	Tea or coffee with sugar	Varies: $\frac{1}{2}$–4+ tsp per cup	8–60+ per cup

* Because of the caffeine in tea and coffee, limit these beverages to no more than four servings per day.

Making such changes can greatly reduce the amount of sugar and calories in your diet, especially for those who tend to drink several sweet sodas or cups of tea and coffee a day. For example, in one year you can save 7,300 teaspoons of sugar or 109,500 calories by eliminating two 12-ounce cans of soda a day. That many extra calories would mean 31 pounds of fat!

tes among Yemenites immigrating there was low. Sucrose is not a part of the traditional diet in Yemen, but the consumption of sucrose by Yemenites immigrating to Israel increased within a short time after their arrival there to the level common in Israel. Within a few years, the Yemenites had a diabetes incidence matching that of other Israelis.

The Israeli investigators, led by A. M. Cohen, M.D., of the Hadassah Medical School in Jerusalem, also undertook laboratory studies and determined that animals on a typically Yemenite, no-sugar diet for 2 months remained normal, while some of those on a western, high-sugar diet developed diabetes symptoms.

The symptomatic animals were probably genetically susceptible. "And this," says Dr. Cohen, "is undoubtedly true of humans. Eating sucrose can bring on diabetes in the genetically prone person. On the other hand, proper dieting—cutting the consumption of refined sugars down to 5 percent of total carbohydrates, not 50—can prevent the onset of diabetes in the genetically prone."

"Currently," Cohen says, "there is no way to tell who is genetically prone to diabetes and who isn't. Therefore, we must all be careful about the consumption of sugar."

Some years ago Dr. Yudkin studied death rates from coronary disease in fifteen countries in relation to sugar intake. The annual coronary death rate per 100,000 persons, he reported, increased steadily from 60 for an intake of 20 pounds of sugar per year to 300 for 120 pounds and then more sharply to about 750 for 150 pounds of sugar per year.

Despite their findings, these and other studies undertaken to date have left many scientists still skeptical about a direct link between sugar consumption and diabetes or coronary heart disease. That doesn't mean, however, that excessive sugar consumption plays no role at all.

Perhaps the views of many scientists are summed up well by Sir Richard Doll, Regius Professor of Medicine at Oxford. "I am not," says Sir Richard, "a believer in the hypothesis that sugar is a specific cause of either. But I think sugar does come into the picture because it makes it easier to eat too much, and if we lower total intake of food, we are more likely to avoid coronary heart disease and diabetes."

Have you been reading a lot about plaque and caries lately and wondering how what you eat influences your dental health? Sugar is the most obvious, and the worst, detriment to

FOOD AND YOUR TEETH

the health of your teeth. Less well-known is the fact that certain other foods, or combinations of foods, can be good or bad for your teeth. For example, although foods rich in fiber are ineffective in removing plaque or harmful food particles, they do stimulate the flow of saliva, which acts as a natural mouthwash. When salivation is suppressed, during sleep or after the use of certain drugs, caries develop more readily.

Plaque is a sticky white substance teeming with bacteria that feed on the bits of food and the residue of sweet drinks that linger in the mouth after eating and drinking. The bacteria produce acid which attacks the enamel surface of teeth, causing them to decay.

Some foods appear to have anticariogenic properties, but others encourage acid production. Some foods, singly or in combination, buffer that acid.

Snack food is often a source of the acid that favors caries production, but that acid can be neutralized if the snacks are eaten with other foods. Here is a list of popular between-meal foods with recommendations about when to enjoy them while protecting your teeth at the same time.

Foods Recommended as Snacks and with Meals

	As snacks	With meals
Fruits	All fresh fruits Unsweetened juices	Dried fruits Pineapples
Vegetables	Raw carrots, celery Cucumbers Lettuce Pickles	All raw or cooked vegetables
Dairy products	Cheeses Plain yogurt Fluid milk	Chocolate-flavored milk Ice cream Sweetened yogurts Milk shakes
Protein products	Nuts Eggs Meats	All meats Beans Peas Peanut butter
Others	Sugar-free gums and candies Soft drinks	Pastries Desserts Regular candies Cookies

SOURCE: Adapted from *Nutrition and Health* 2(3):5, 1980.

Cariogenic Sweeteners and Their Sources

Sugar	Natural sources	Used in
Sucrose	Found in large amounts in:	
	Sugar cane	Soft drinks
	Sugar beets	Pastries
	Maple syrup	Candies
	Molasses	Chewing gums
	Fruits	Desserts
	Found in moderate amounts in:	
	Vegetables	Ready-to-eat cereals
Glucose	Found in moderate amounts in:	
	Honey	Pancake syrup
	Corn syrup	
	Found in small amounts in:	
	Fruits	
	Vegetables	
	Grains*	
	Legumes*	
	Tubers*	
Fructose	Found in large amounts in:	
	Honey	
	Found in moderate amounts in:	
	Fruits	Table syrup
	Vegetables	Candies
Lactose	Found in:	
	Milk	

* In the form of starch.
SOURCE: *Nutrition and Health* 2(3):4, 1980.

Noncariogenic Sweeteners and Their Sources

Sweetener	Natural source	Used in
Xylitol	Many plants	Chewing gum
	Commercially produced from wood	
Sorbitol	Fruits	Dietetic products
	Vegetables	Chewing gums
	Commercially produced from sugar	Mints
		Pharmaceuticals
Mannitol	Manna ash tree	Chewing gums
	Seaweed	Dietetic products
	Commercially produced from sugar	
Saccharin	Commercially produced from coal tar	Soft drinks
		Pharmaceuticals
		Tooth paste
		Dietetic products

Adding It All Up

The important points in this chapter can be summarized as follows.

Carbohydrates

These are ready energy sources, easily converted by the body to glucose. Glucose can be readily oxidized (burned) to produce carbon dioxide, water, heat, and energy. If not needed for immediate energy, glucose can be stored as glycogen or fat.

Not all carbohydrates are equal in value.

* To be encouraged: *intake of cereals, breads, potatoes, and other fruits and vegetables which contain carbohydrates and, in addition, vitamins, minerals, and proteins.*

* To be discouraged: *excess intake of foods high in refined sugar (sucrose), which contains calories but few nutrients.*

Carbohydrates spare protein. Given enough carbohydrates, the body does not have to utilize large amounts of protein for energy, so the protein can serve its primary function of tissue maintenance and repair.

Inadequate dietary carbohydrates, in addition to failing to spare protein, can cause the body to make use of fat as a major energy source. With excess use of fat for that purpose, there may be an accumulation in the body of the potentially toxic breakdown products of fat.

Fats

Fats can be used to provide energy, or, if not needed immediately for that purpose, they can be stored for later use.

Excessive fat intake is not desirable. It may cause obesity, heart disease, and other problems.

Many authorities urge a reduction of fat intake. The American Heart Association suggests that it be limited to 30 to 35 percent of total calories. The Senate Select Committee on Nutrition and Human Needs calls for a maximum of 30 percent. Recently, the American Diabetes Association has encouraged diabetics to limit fat (particularly of animal origin) in their daily diet.

This is best achieved by replacing foods high in fat with more whole-grain breads, fruits, and vegetables, by using skim milk instead of whole milk, by eating more chicken and fish instead of fatty meats, and by using vegetable oils in place of other fats for cooking.

Proteins

During digestion, proteins are broken down into their constituent amino acids, which the body then reconstitutes in the various combinations needed for its functions.

If overall energy requirements are not being met—if there is inadequate carbohydrate or fat in the diet—the body turns protein into glucose or fat for energy. Protein deficiency may result.

When protein intake exceeds actual needs, the excess is turned into sugar or fat and stored.

The Interacting System

The body can get the energy it needs from the daily diet or from its stored supply (mainly fat). When more energy is available than is immediately needed, the body conserves it, storing it away as fat for later use.

Fat is not readily broken down for energy; glucose is needed if it is to be used effectively. The body keeps some glucose in storage as glycogen in the liver and muscles, but this reserve is limited. It can only last about 16 hours without being replenished by the consumption of carbohydrates.

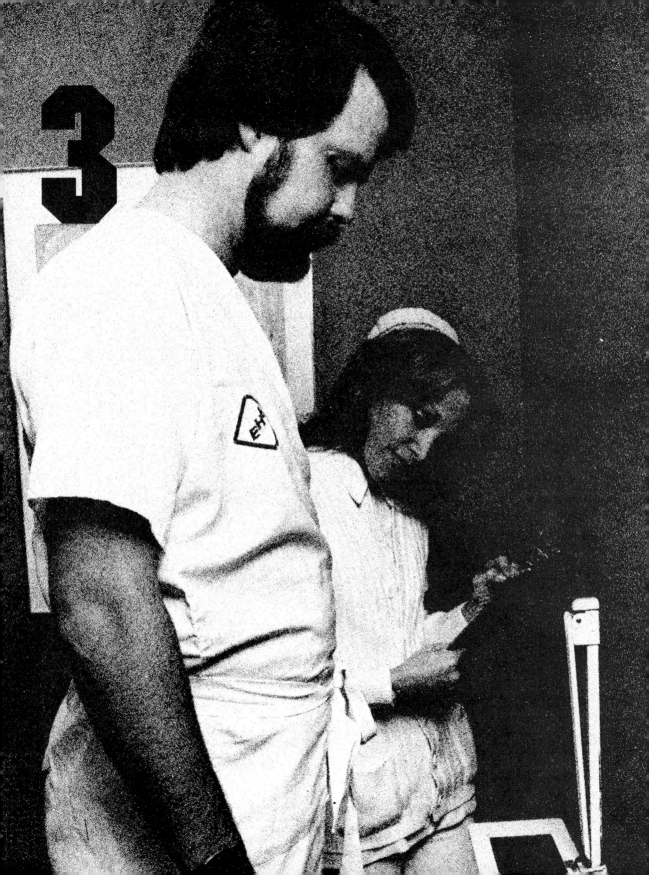

3

NUTRITION AND WEIGHT CONTROL

If you're overweight, you're ill.

"If you're overweight, you're ill. And I mean seriously ill. Oh, that's not to say you won't get away with it for a long time. Or that you won't feel perfectly well. . . . But in the end, the fat will get you."

So wrote physician Robert E. Fuiz some years ago.

His reasons: "Carrying extra weight batters your arteries, plunders your heart, predisposes you to diabetes, and pounds away at the weight-bearing joints so that in the end a fat man wobbles where a thin man runs. It's sad, really. . . . Being fat is being sick. Honest."

The Obesity Epidemic

In the United States today, it is a rare person who does not diet or does not know someone else who diets. At any given moment, some 20 million Americans are on one kind of diet or another. Although women have been the mainstay of the diet industry, men are becoming increasingly concerned about their weight, too.

About 40 percent of all Americans, it is estimated, are at least 20 percent above their ideal weight. For some age groups, including men from 38 to 48 and women from 50 to 60, the figure is 65 percent.

The Bad News

Although there must be a thousand or more programs to help people lose weight in what has become a leading minor growth industry at $10 billion a year, the record of success in losing and keeping off weight is abysmal.

Writing in the specialty journal, *Obesity & Bariatric Medicine*, Margaret Mackenzie, M.D., observes: "Losing weight is easy; keeping it off is impossible for more than about two percent of those who try. Two years later, almost all who have successfully lost weight have not only regained it, but added more as well."

Ironically, Americans, generally considered the most diet-conscious people on earth, are not getting thinner, as the Metropolitan Life Insurance Company discovered when it conducted a study of its policyholders going back 30 years. Over that time period, the average weight for men increased by 11 pounds, from 160 to 171 pounds, and the average weight for women rose by 5 pounds, from 129 to 134 pounds.

OBESITY IN PERSPECTIVE

"Obesity—many of us die younger because of it, suffer a number of associated physical ailments because of it, spend great amounts of money trying to get rid of it, and understand very little about it. Obesity is a chronic American affliction."

RoseAnn Shorey, M.D., University of Texas

"Nearly every form of cancer has a higher cure rate than does obesity. Many studies indicate that obesity tends to be chronic and that most individuals who lose weight will regain it. Successful weight programs, therefore, must be aimed at assisting the patient to maintain weight loss through establishing *a lifetime eating style which ensures good nutrition without excess calories*" [italics added].

Mary B. McCann, M.D., Massachusetts Mental Health Center

The Good News

In spite of depressing statistics, obesity is not incurable—far from it. There is nothing inherently insurmountable about it.

What does seem to be insurmountable is the misguided faith placed by so many people in fad diets, in the latest

The record of success in losing and keeping off weight is abysmal.

"quickie" panaceas, which rarely, if ever, do more than make their inventors rich.

Precisely because they result in quick losses of weight and do not permanently substitute good eating and drinking habits for poor ones, fad diets seldom achieve stable weight loss.

However, for the executive who is determined to achieve it, stable weight loss is possible. We know that from our experience at Executive Health Examiners.

We know, too, from our experience that the achievement can be far less burdensome than many people think—and clearly worth the effort, as C.M., a vice president in charge of operations for a large conglomerate, found out.

C.M. was 60 pounds over his ideal weight. He blamed this on occupational stress and the fact that he traveled 3 or 4 days of every week throughout the United States.

At Executive Health Examiners, the nutritionist determined that because C.M. was a very motivated, goal-oriented, and disciplined person, he would stick to the 1800-calorie exchange-type diet that was prescribed. The diet offered a wide variety of food selected from each food group, so even though his lifestyle included so much travel, C.M. was able to stay on the diet while working, at business lunches, at home, and on social occasions.

A stress test given by an EHE physician showed that C.M. would be a good candidate for an exercise program, which would provide an opportunity for stress reduction as well as for additional weight loss. The nutritionist helped him select practical exercises that would not tax his busy time schedule. Now he travels with a jump rope, climbs hotel and office stairs, and walks briskly for a half-hour or more each day. Because he was highly motivated, C.M. lost weight within 6

Obesity is not incurable — far from it.

months and has assumed a lifestyle that will allow him to maintain his new, lower weight through continued exercise and prudent eating.

The Penalties of Obesity

The stereotype of the jolly fat person may be the most inaccurate myth in American culture. Perhaps Cyril Connolly

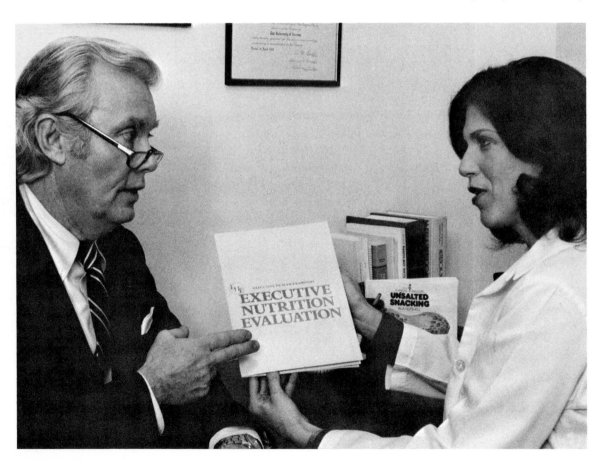

came closer to the truth when he said, "Inside every fat person, there is a thin person, screaming to be let out."

Beyond whatever psychological discomforts it may cause, obesity is associated with health hazards, among them the following.

Breathing Difficulties The greater the weight in the chest wall, the greater the work involved in breathing. Because of their increased breathing difficulty, obese people have less tolerance for exercise.

Coronary Heart Disease Excess weight is a risk factor for coronary heart disease and the heart attacks which that disease may produce. In the government's long-term Framingham Heart Study, which has been following more than 5000 originally healthy people in that Massachusetts community for more than 30 years, men who were 30 percent overweight turned out to have a 2.8 times greater risk of developing coronary heart disease within 10 years of their becoming that overweight than those who were 10 percent or more underweight during the same period of time. Obesity may promote coronary heart disease because it adds to the burden of the heart, which must provide circulation for the extra fatty tissue. Blood-fat abnormalities also are more common among the obese.

High Blood Pressure The blood pressure of the obese is often elevated. High blood pressure contributes to coronary heart disease and is also a major factor in stroke and kidney disease.

Gallbladder Disease Obesity is associated with increased production of cholesterol and, hence, with increased concentration of cholesterol in bile, which is pro-

The stereotype of the jolly fat person may be the most inaccurate myth in American culture.

duced in the liver and stored in the gallbladder. If the concentration of cholesterol becomes great enough, the cholesterol may precipitate out of the bile as gallstones.

Diabetes Obesity is clearly related to the most common form of diabetes mellitus—adult-onset diabetes. Obesity, research indicates, seems to lead to resistance to the action of insulin, which normally transfers glucose (blood sugar) to the body tissues.

Weight Reduction Effects

Gratifyingly, many studies have demonstrated that eliminating excess weight helps significantly to reduce elevated levels of blood fats (cholesterol and triglycerides), to reduce elevated blood pressure, and to decrease insulin resistance.

S.D. is a busy executive who agreed to measures that may have saved his life. At 57, he was the personnel director of a large company, and never had a moment to spare. He had never paid much attention to his weight, which was 35

PRINCIPAL CAUSES OF DEATH AMONG THE OBESE*

	Male	Female
Cardiovascular/ renal disease	149	177
Stroke	159	162
Diabetes	383	372
Chronic kidney disease	191	212
Cancer: Liver/gallbladder	168	211
Breast		69
Gallstones	152	188
Cirrhosis of liver	249	147
Appendicitis	223	195

* Death rates of persons accepted for standard insurance = 100% actual of expected deaths.

The right diet and exercise at the right time probably saved S.D. from a heart attack or the need for coronary bypass surgery.

pounds above normal or to his cholesterol level, which was 320 milligrams per deciliter of blood serum (the normal range is 120 to 250 milligrams per deciliter). He had always felt "great" until the past year, when he developed chest pains while walking to work. After a stress test, the physician told S.D. he had angina pectoris and prescribed appropriate medication for him. S.D. was not happy about this and, moreover, felt only partial relief from the pain.

As an adjunct to the medication, the physician prescribed a modified exercise program and sent S.D. to the EHE nutritionist for a low-calorie, low-cholesterol diet. Within 7 months he lost weight and lowered his serum cholesterol level, and his angina symptoms disappeared almost completely. His medication was subsequently reduced by more than half.

The right diet and exercise at the right time probably saved S.D. from a heart attack or the need for coronary bypass surgery.

"THE LARGEST BIOLOGICAL STUDY EVER UNDERTAKEN OF LIFE AND DEATH"

The recently reported American Cancer Society study, which has been given that appellation, may well deserve it. It was huge and long-term. Some 68,000 volunteer workers for the society enrolled more than 1 million men and women in the study. Every year over the following 12 years, the volunteers reported if the enrolled individuals were alive or dead. If an enrollee had died, a copy of the death certificate was obtained.

At the end of 12 years, 92.8 percent of the study population (alive or dead) had been successfully traced. The data were analyzed to determine the variations in mortality by weight among the 336,442 men and 419,060 women who were traced through the course of the study, and who were not ill on entry into the survey and had had no history of cancer, heart disease, or stroke.

Mortality steadily increased with overweight. If average-weight mortality is taken to be 100, the mortality rate was 115 for men at 110 to 119 percent of average weight, 127 at 120 to 129 percent of average weight, 146 at 130 to 139 percent of average weight, and 187 over 140 percent of average weight. For women, the corresponding mortality rates were 117, 127, 146, and 189.

When mortality rates in the overweight were analyzed by diseases (again considering mortality for a disease in the average-weight category as 100), the rates in the most overweight groups of men were 519 for diabetes, 399 for digestive diseases, 227 for cerebrovascular disease, 195 for coronary heart disease, and 133 for cancer. For women, the corresponding figures were 790, 299, 152, 207, and 155.

Without any doubt, overweight people of both sexes tend to die sooner than their lean contemporaries.

Are You Obese?

By definition, an obese person is one who weighs 20 percent or more than what he or she should weigh.

Even if you are not obese, it may still be worthwhile for you to lose 10 pounds or so of whatever excess weight you are carrying. Chances are that if you are overweight at all, you will gain more weight in the future, and it is easier to lose 10 pounds now than 20, 30, 50, or more pounds in the future. Here are some easy ways of checking on your weight.

Overweight people tend to die sooner than their lean contemporaries.

The Mirror Test Usually, your mirror can provide you with a fairly good clue to whether you are too heavy. Remove all your clothes and take a look—back, side, and front—in a full-length mirror. Stop holding your breath and sucking in your gut. Examine the real you.

Desirable-Weight Chart Consult the table on page 56 to determine if your eyes have deceived you. Note that this table, unlike some others, gives "desirable" rather than "average" weights. What is "average" tends to include more and more fat as you progress from age group to age group, and

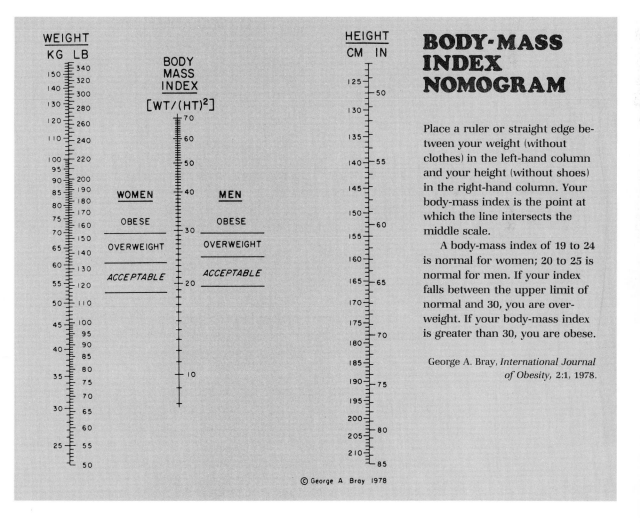

BODY-MASS INDEX NOMOGRAM

Place a ruler or straight edge between your weight (without clothes) in the left-hand column and your height (without shoes) in the right-hand column. Your body-mass index is the point at which the line intersects the middle scale.

A body-mass index of 19 to 24 is normal for women; 20 to 25 is normal for men. If your index falls between the upper limit of normal and 30, you are overweight. If your body-mass index is greater than 30, you are obese.

George A. Bray, *International Journal of Obesity*, 2:1, 1978.

© George A Bray 1978

DESIRABLE WEIGHTS BY HEIGHT FOR ADULT MALES AND FEMALES*

Height without shoes		Weight without clothes			
		Men		Women	
in	cm	lb	kg	lb	kg
58	147			102 (92–119)	46 (42–54)
60	152			107 (96–125)	49 (44–57)
62	158	123 (112–141)	56 (51–64)	113 (102–131)	51 (46–59)
64	163	130 (118–148)	59 (54–67)	120 (108–138)	55 (49–63)
66	168	136 (124–156)	62 (56–71)	128 (114–146)	58 (52–66)
68	173	145 (132–166)	66 (60–75)	136 (122–154)	62 (55–70)
70	178	154 (140–174)	70 (64–79)	144 (130–163)	65 (59–74)
72	183	162 (148–184)	74 (67–84)	152 (138–173)	69 (63–79)
74	188	171 (156–194)	78 (71–88)		
76	193	181 (164–204)	82 (74–93)		

* Average weight ranges in parentheses.
SOURCE: George A. Bray, 1975.

that is *not* desirable. Also, average-weight tables reflect the weight of overweight individuals, who skew the average upward.

The Pinch Test Grasp a fold of skin with your thumb and forefinger—at your waist, stomach, upper arm, buttocks, and calf. At least half of body fat is directly under the skin. Generally, the under-skin layer (which is what you measure with the pinch, since only fat, not muscle, pinches) should be between $\frac{1}{4}$ and $\frac{1}{2}$ inch thick. Since you get a double thickness with your pinch, it normally should be $\frac{1}{2}$ to 1 inch. A fold much greater than an inch indicates excess body fat.

The Ruler Test This test is based on the fact that if there is no excess fat, the abdominal surface—between the flare of the ribs and the front of the pelvis—normally is flat. If you lie on your back and place a ruler on your abdomen, along the midline of the body, it should not point upward at the midsection. If your stomach holds up the ruler so it doesn't lie flat, you need to slim down.

A simple rule of thumb by which a woman can determine her ideal weight is to begin with a base weight of 100 pounds for 5 feet of height and add 5 pounds for each inch by which she is taller than 5 feet. This will give the ideal weight for an average body frame. For a woman 5 feet 4 inches tall, the ideal weight is 120 pounds. For a small body frame, subtract 10 percent from the total; for a large body frame, add 10 percent.

Men should begin with a base weight of 106 pounds for 5 feet of height and add 6 pounds for each inch by which they are taller than 5 feet. The same allowances can be used for body frame difference. So the ideal weight for a 5-foot 10-inch man of average build is 166 pounds.

To figure your basal calorie need (how many calories you burn up when at complete rest), just add a zero to your ideal weight. If your ideal weight is 166 pounds, you need at least 1660 calories a day to maintain your weight.

How does your basal calorie need compare with your actual total daily calorie need? If you live a sedentary life, add a third again onto the basal calorie need. If you are athletic—say, if you run or jog 5 miles a day—you can take in twice your basal requirement and still maintain your weight. If you are moderately active, getting about 90 minutes of exercise a week, add half again to your basal calorie requirement.

Factors that Contribute to Obesity

Obesity can have many contributing causes, one or more of which may predominate in a given individual. Some of those causes are well-established; research is turning up others.

Genetic Predisposition

That a hereditary influence—a genetic predisposition—can be at work in some cases of obesity has been shown by studies of obese identical twins. Some were raised together; others, apart. Despite environmental differences, both groups tended to become obese.

Still environment is influential too. Studies have shown that genetically predisposed youngsters raised by nonobese adoptive parents do not become as obese as predisposed youngsters placed in families with obese adoptive parents. Also, children who are not genetically predisposed to obesity tend to be heavier when raised by obese adoptive parents than nonpredisposed children raised by nonobese adoptive parents.

Fat Children and Fat Cells

Many of us become obese only in adulthood, but others get an early start, even in the first months of life. The latter can be the particularly unlucky ones—fat in the sandbox, fat through school, fat now, and facing a very tough fight if they are not to die fat.

One reason for their difficulty is an excess of fat cells, tiny structures that are located throughout the body, with large concentrations in the abdomen and around such organs as the kidneys and the heart.

We all have such cells, which collect and hold fat from food intake, keeping it in storage for use when needed. Whether we all have the same number at birth is unknown. However, two facts about the cells have become known recently. One is that once a fat cell appears in the body, it remains for a lifetime, although the amount of fat stored in any given cell can vary from day to day and from year to year.

The second fact is that the number of these permanent fat cells can multiply—doubling or even tripling—in the first months of life. Such multiplication, it appears, can cause problems. The baby fed moderately so that no such multiplication occurs is far less likely to have trouble with obesity throughout life than the infant fed too much and thereafter burdened with an excess of fat cells.

Many of us become obese only in adulthood, but others get an early start, even in the first months of life.

Studying obese children, Jerome Knittle, M.D., of Mt. Sinai School of Medicine, New York City, removed small amounts of tissue from under the skin with a special syringe. He found 2-year-old obese children with double the number of fat cells of normal-weight children of the same age and 5-year-olds with more fat cells than normal adults.

There is some evidence that excess fat cells may communicate with the appetite center in the brain, signaling a need to be filled. An overabundance of such cells, then, may lead to excessive appetite.

Physical Inactivity

Many studies of both children and adults have shown that the obese commonly are less active than the lean. Interestingly, too, studies of people who have deliberately eaten to excess in order to become obese have shown that physical activity tends to decrease as obesity increases.

Glandular Disorders

In some cases, endocrine gland disorders can play a significant role in obesity. Underfunctioning of the thyroid gland (hypothyroidism) can make weight loss difficult unless it is corrected. Rarely, disorders of other glands—the adrenals, pancreas, or pituitary—may contribute to obesity. However, glandular dysfunction is considered by most authorities to be highly overrated as a cause of obesity; it is responsible at most for no more than 1 percent of excess weight.

The "Habit Belly"

Virtually all of us do some eating without hunger, but many of the obese far surpass us. They often eat in large measure because of environmental cues—time of day, odors, palatability of food, sight of food. They may nibble without thinking while reading or watching television. They may eat simply because it is mealtime, and they may finish everything in front of them even though they are not hungry. They commonly eat when feeling depressed, bored, or lonesome.

This is learned behavior. It may be learned even in early childhood. Newborns naturally react to hunger pangs by sucking on breast or bottle until they feel comfortably full; then they stop. Even during infancy, however, external clues may intrude and trigger eating. If parents praise their children for finishing their bottles, the children may come to do some of their eating thereafter not out of hunger but in seeking praise. If children are given sweets to comfort them when they fall and hurt themselves, they may be learning to assuage pain—both physical and emotional—with food. And parents who give their children crackers or cookies to ease teething pain may be leading them into the habit of eating without being hungry.

A New Possibility—An Enzyme Defect

A biochemical defect that changes the way the body burns food for energy may result in a predisposition toward obesity, according to Harvard Medical School researchers Mario DeLuise, Jeffrey Flier, and George Blackburn. Their discovery suggests that some people with weight problems may burn up fewer calories for energy than do normal people and may store more calories as fat.

Obese people, the investigators found, have a significantly lower level of an enzyme which helps to chemically balance the internal and external environments of cells. Called the *sodium-potassium-pump*, adenosine triphosphatase (ATPase) is an enzyme which transports sodium and potassium across the membrane of every living cell, keeping sodium levels low and potassium levels high.

In its work, ATPase uses from 20 to 50 percent of each day's food intake and generates heat as a by-product, thereby sustaining normal body temperature. Overweight people, suggest the investigators, may expend far less energy to maintain the sodium-potassium balance than do people of average weight.

They studied twenty overweight (47 to 177 percent higher than ideal weight) adult volunteers and twenty others with normal weights. The obese subjects were found to have a markedly lower level of ATPase in their red blood cells, and the heavier the individual, the lower the level.

The ATPase discovery may have significance beyond the understanding of weight gain.

The researchers now plan to go beyond red blood cells and study ATPase in other body tissues of obese and normal people. They hope to learn which hormones regulate the enzyme levels and whether age has anything to do with varying levels.

The ATPase discovery may have significance beyond understanding weight gain. The enzyme plays a role in other biological processes, and if the blood-cell abnormality is also found in other body cells, it may be linked to disorders common in overweight people, such as hypertension and diabetes.

One approach to further investigation would be to study certain groups of people genetically predisposed to both obesity and diabetes. Arizona's Pima Indians, for example, endured centuries of feast-and-famine cycles in the past, and their survival may have depended on their ability to maintain bodily reserves in the form of excess fat. Today, despite food supplies that are more certain, their bodies continue to store excess fat for famines that never come.

HAVE YOU EVER SEEN A FAT TIGER?

With only a few notable exceptions, such as overindulged house pets and special obese strains of mice, humans are the only beings on earth with a weight problem. In the wild, obesity is virtually nonexistent.

The reason for our obesity, suggests George Cahill, M.D., Harvard Medical School, is that at one time it may have been an advantage for some of our ancestors to be able to override an internal signal that told them not to overeat—and some of us have lost touch with the signal.

Experiments have shown a precisely calibrated biological feedback mechanism that lets animals know exactly how much they need to eat to go about their daily business.

In one study, the subject was a 300-gram female rat. When her food was taken away, she lost weight. When food was reintroduced, she ate right back up to 300 grams and no more—"without the benefit of a rat scale," observed Dr. Cahill.

Then her food was cut with some noncaloric material so that the pellets contained only half the original number of calories. Promptly, she ate twice as much food as before—"because," says Cahill, "she knows she should weigh 300 grams."

Human studies have shown the presence of a similar mechanism, but in human beings it can be disturbed by psychological, environmental, or biological factors.

During the 1960s, a group of young male prisoners volunteered to test a synthetic liquid diet developed for NASA. At the end of a week it turned out that all the subjects were drinking 8 to 10 cans a day—2400 to 3000 calories, exactly the amount of energy they were expending.

According to Dr. Cahill, "There was something in these kids that said, 'Look, you're supposed to eat just this amount of calories per day.'"

In another study, male college students were put on a diet of milk shakes. Without their knowledge, some got genuine milk shakes with real ice cream and 300 to 400 calories while others got a variety made with artificial sweetener and nonnutritive bulk, containing only about 100 calories. Nevertheless, both groups took in remarkably similar numbers of calories; those getting the ersatz preparation drank more of it.

Both studies were done with young subjects. Dr. Cahill reports that in most young people, particularly thinner ones, body weight rarely changes very much from week to week or month to month, but the caloric regulator seems to disappear around the third decade of life, suggesting that the biological feedback mechanism may begin to malfunction at this point.

Fad Diets and Diet Pills

Dieting has been called the number one national pastime, and fad diets have been referred to as "true pollutants of national health."

New diets appear almost weekly and are followed—

often one right after the other—always with hope, however bizarre, self-defeating, and even health-impairing they may be.

"Magic Pair" Diets and Crash Diets

"Magic Pair" diets, such as the Beverly Hills diet, claim to produce quick weight loss if you eat only certain pairs of foods, such as grapefruit and lamb chops, eggs and spinach, or bananas and skim milk. On a crash diet, you may eat nothing but grapefruit and drink nothing but water, or you may only eat celery and drink water, or you may eat only cottage cheese, or something similar. While the idea of both kinds of diet is to melt away a lot of fat in little time, the actual effect is to make the dieter miserable and place him or her at risk of malnutrition. Also, fat that is quickly lost is usually quickly regained.

High-Protein Diets

These are diets which restrict food intake to steak, eggs, and other high-protein foods. Any diet restricted to a single category of foods is dangerous because it omits other necessary food groups. High-protein diets are also high in animal fat, salt, and cholesterol. They leave out essential nutrients that come from fresh fruits and vegetables.

"Eat Fat" Diets

Supposedly, this kind of diet puts the fats you eat to work, somehow miraculously melting away fat deposits in the body. Americans have spent millions of dollars on books advocating such diets. There is no evidence whatever that any one type of food has special value in stimulating the burning off of fat stores.

Low-Carbohydrate Diets

A diet sometimes called the Air Force Diet is one of many such diets, but it is vigorously disclaimed by the Air Force. It calls for restricting the intake of "carbohydrate units" but allows you to eat anything else you want. However, carbohydrate restriction may upset digestion and impair body fluid balance. Carbohydrates, moreover, are needed to help metabolize fats; in their absence a dangerous condition called *ketosis* may develop as fat metabolism becomes incomplete and products of the incomplete metabolism accumulate in the blood. Furthermore, low-carbohydrate diets tend to concentrate on foods high in fats, especially saturated fats, which may be harmful to the coronary arteries.

There are endless variations on these diets, purveyed under eye-catching new names in countless magazine articles and books. But however attractive their claims may sound, they are self-defeating, even when they are not outright dangerous. They may appear to be successful initially in removing weight, but the initial weight loss is due to water loss (rather than loss of body fat) and/or a decrease in appetite and thus in calorie intake. Because of the radical change in eating habits dictated by these diets, no one can, or should, continue on them for a long time. Also, as old eating practices are resumed, weight lost on these diets is quickly regained.

It may be worthwhile to examine two of the most popular diets of recent years.

Dr. Atkins' Diet This is one more version of the high-fat type of diet. As far back as 1864, when his "Letter on Corpulence" was published, William Banting, coffin maker to the Duke of Wellington, espoused such a diet. It has appeared under other names since, including the Du Pont Diet, which was in vogue in the early 1950s.

Followers of this diet eat no carbohydrates during the first week—no fruits, vegetables, or breads. They can, however, eat as much as they want of bacon and eggs, marbled steaks, and the like. The high intake of fat from eating such foods leads to ketosis as substances called *ketone bodies* (incompletely burned fat) appear. In the second phase of this diet, very small amounts of carbohydrates are gradually added to the diet as long as ketosis continues.

The Atkins diet has been attacked as a "bizarre regimen" and one "without scientific merit" by the American Medical

Association's Council on Foods and Nutrition and as "unbalanced, unsound and unsafe" by *The Medical Letter.*

Among the criticisms voiced against the Atkins diet are the following:

* *The consumption of large amounts of saturated fats can raise the blood cholesterol level and contribute to coronary heart disease.*

* *Ketosis, which physicians consider to be an abnormal metabolic state, can damage the kidneys and alter the normal acid-alkaline balance.*

* *Very low carbohydrate intake can lead to fatigue, apathy, nausea, and heart irregularities.*

* *Most of the weight lost with very low carbohydrate intake is due to loss of water and is quickly regained.*

* *This is not a diet with which one can live comfortably for a lifetime.*

The Scarsdale Medical Group Diet   This diet is said to be based on chemical reactions between foods and is said to maintain normal energy levels while resulting in weight losses of up to 20 pounds in 14 days.

Almost all carbohydrates and significant amounts of fat are forbidden. Only lean meats are allowed. All foods must be prepared without butter, and all salads without oil or mayonnaise. No substitutions, no alcohol, and no between-meal snacks are allowed, except for raw carrots and celery. No one is supposed to stay on the diet for more than 14 days at a time.

The Scarsdale diet has been criticized on the grounds that it is unbalanced and too high in protein. Since it is low in calories, it will lead to weight loss, but because it is unbalanced, it must be abandoned after a short time, with rapid weight gain inevitable as the dieter returns to previous eating patterns.

For a busy executive who entertains frequently or who enjoys socializing with friends over meals at restaurants or

The Scarsdale diet has been criticized on the grounds that it is unbalanced and too high in protein.

at home, the diet (with its lack of choices and substitutions) is not practical.

Diet Pills—Are They of Any Value?

To many people, the true wonder drug would be one that could melt away fat, making weight control entirely effortless, but it simply is not available nor is it ever likely to be. However, there are many drugs that have been used for this purpose.

Amphetamines For a while some years ago, amphetamines were claimed to be valuable as appetite suppressants, and in fact, those who took them felt less hunger. Then serious side effects were recognized, including increased blood pressure and heart rate, drug dependency, and bouts of depression when the pills were withdrawn.

Amphetamine-like Agents There are a number of other appetite-suppressant drugs, such as diethylpropion and phentermine, that are available for physicians to prescribe. Almost all are derivatives of amphetamine.

Tolerance develops in a few weeks, so they lose their effectiveness unless potentially dangerous large doses are taken. These drugs can be habit-forming. Among the adverse reactions to them are palpitations, elevation of blood pressure, restlessness, insomnia, tremor, headache, hives, and impotence.

Some 200 studies of amphetamine-like agents recently reviewed by the Food and Drug Administration indicate that taking such drugs results in only an extra half pound of weight loss per week. As some authorities point out, since tolerance develops and drug makers therefore suggest only a short course of 2 to 4 weeks, the average added benefit of appetite suppressants is only 1 to 2 pounds of weight loss— hardly worth the risks they entail.

Diuretics These prescription agents have no real value in weight control. They only promote excretion of water, with no effect on fat, and the water is replaced promptly when use of the drug is stopped. Indiscriminate use of diuretics can upset the body's mineral balance, leading to serious losses of sodium and potassium. They may also cause nausea, weakness, and dizziness.

Thyroid Compounds These speed up metabolism and may lead to some weight loss. But, except in persons who actually need them because of low thyroid function, thyroid compounds can produce hyperthyroid symptoms such as irritability, diarrhea, and abnormal heart rhythms.

Nonprescription Products These contain one or the other of two agents: benzocaine or phenylpropanolamine.

Benzocaine, a local anesthetic sometimes used to soothe

THE CURRENT AMERICAN DIET AND GOALS FOR ITS IMPROVEMENT

Current diet*	Dietary goals
42% fat:	30% fat:
16% saturated fat	10% saturated fat
19% monounsaturated fat	10% monounsaturated fat
7% polyunsaturated fat	10% polyunsaturated fat
12% protein	12% protein
46% carbohydrates:	58% carbohydrates:
22% complex carbohydrates	48% complex carbohydrates and
6% naturally occurring sugars†	naturally occurring sugars
18% refined and processed sugars‡	10% refined and processed sugars

* These percentages are based on calories from food and nonalcoholic beverages.
† *Naturally occurring* denotes sugars which are indigenous to a food as opposed to refined (cane and beet) and processed (corn sugar, syrups, molasses, and honey) sugars which may be added to a food product.
‡ In many ways alcoholic beverages affect the diet in the same way as refined and other processed sugars. Both add calories (energy) to the total diet but contribute little or no vitamins or minerals.
SOURCE: Senate Select Committee on Nutrition and Human Needs.

skin irritations, can be found in special chewing gums or candy. It is supposed to dull the taste buds and discourage eating.

Phenylpropanolamine (PPA), an amphetamine-related drug which has been used as a nasal decongestant in cold remedies, can be found in popular diet pills such as Dexatrim, Prolaine, Spantrol, and Appedrine. The drug is supposed to depress the appetite center in the brain. It has been found to elevate blood pressure in normal subjects.

Drug companies warn against use of these drugs by people with high blood pressure, diabetes, diseases of the heart, kidney, or thyroid, or other diseases. Such conditions often afflict the overweight, in many instances without their knowledge. The drugs also should not be used during pregnancy.

Even if they did no harm, do these drugs do much good?

No. At best they may serve as a temporary crutch. The phenylpropanolamine and benzocaine preparations that you can buy without a prescription are to be used for strictly limited periods—no longer than 3 months.

For long-term weight control, they are completely useless.

There wasn't a fad diet that B.R. hadn't tried at least once in his life—grapefruit and eggs, tuna blitz, Atkins, and Stillman—besides having taken diuretics, laxatives, and diet pills. He had tried everything to lose weight over the past 40 years, ever since he was in high school.

B.R., 56 years old and a successful businessman, was only 10 pounds overweight when he made his first visit to the EHE dietician. He admitted, however, that his weight went up and down 10 pounds at least five times each year— what we at Executive Health Examiners call the "yo-yo" pattern of weight control. He also recognized that such fluctuation is not good for a person's health. B.R.'s latest effort to follow a popular "movie-star fruit-only" diet had ended when he fainted one evening at home and hit his head on a piece of furniture.

He felt desperate. "Please put me on a very strict diet with no substitutions," he pleaded. "I don't do well when I'm given choices." The nutritionist refused to contribute to further failure by instituting yet another fad diet. She gave

A QUICK BREAK FOR LUNCH

"If I'm working and want to break for 15 or 20 minutes for lunch, I can stop in a deli and get a turkey sandwich on rye bread, with maybe a little tomato and zucchini salad with vinaigrette dressing, and a glass of Perrier, which is a pretty healthy lunch.

"Or I can go two blocks the other way and grab a cheeseburger and order of fries, and an apple turnover for dessert.

"I have that choice. Both are equally quick. Each contains nutrients, but the second choice adds salt, cholesterol, and more calories."

An EHE physician

MASSAGES AND HOT BATHS

Massage does not help take off fat. Once the fat is off, however, massage may tone up the skin and muscles and help the body adjust to its new, slimmer contours.

The effect of hot baths lasts very briefly. They serve only to eliminate some water, which almost immediately is regained. In addition to being useless for permanent weight reduction, these methods can put a strain on the heart and circulation. Sauna baths, for example, expose the body to high temperatures and produce violent sweating—a shock to the body—sometimes doubling the pulse rate. Saunas have long been popular in Finland; however, the Finns use them over a lifetime rather than starting suddenly in flabby middle age. Saunas do little for obesity.

B.R. a food diary and insisted that he should eat anything he wanted for the next 2 weeks, as long as he wrote it down.

B.R. made a discovery that was surprising (to him at least) —his eating habits were not as bad as he had imagined. With a few modifications of diet and behavior, plus increased exercise, B.R. has achieved a true weight-control program for the first time in his life. Now he follows a normal diet and has never felt better.

Effective Weight Control

Effective weight control means more than just losing weight; it means maintaining the reduced weight permanently. That can be achieved with a sound diet based on your current eating habits—nothing extreme, nothing bizarre, and nothing to place your health at risk.

Permanent weight reduction is more likely to be

Effective weight control means more than just losing weight.

achieved—and more readily achievable without strain—if a diet is coupled with physical activity that increases energy expenditure—and in the process makes other contributions to health.

The likelihood of success is also markedly increased by behavior-modification techniques that change inappropriate eating habits, many of which can be altered quite easily.

L.P., a 39-year-old public relations executive who had worked her way up to a prime position in her company, proved to be a good candidate for this approach, although the changes did not happen all at once.

L.P. considers personal appearance to be an important aspect of her job; nevertheless, she has been 25 pounds overweight for most of her adult life. When she was 25, she attended a popular weight-control group and lost her excess weight on their regimented program, but she regained it all within several months and since then has felt very discouraged.

When L.P. visited the nutritionist at Executive Health Examiners and expressed her discouragement, the nutritionist helped her define her goal—to lose the 25 pounds of extra weight very gradually without feeling deprived. For the next year, L.P. worked closely with the nutritionist. Because it was important to her to be in control of her dietary decisions, just as she was in control of the rest of her life, a system of compromises was established for excess calories and portion sizes, as well as a behavior-modification plan. No regimented dietary plan was designed.

After L.P. had lost 15 pounds, she hit a "plateau" and was unable to lose any more weight for 3 months. She returned to the EHE nutritionist, who helped her to identify the problem. A woman accustomed to achieving, L.P. was fearful of failure. She was afraid she would repeat her experience and return to her obese condition. After much encouragement from the nutritionist, she was convinced that this totally new approach of modifying her existing eating behavior patterns would bring lasting success, not failure. L.P. lost the additional 10 pounds and has maintained this loss for 3 years.

The Exercise Factor

For years, the role of exercise in weight control has been commonly misunderstood, but today regular physical activity is known to be important for maintaining health and preventing many diseases.

As for weight control, it can be said that while diet is part of the battle and helps you on your way, exercise contributes vitality and drive and helps take you where you want to go.

Looking at exercise recently, the U.S. Surgeon General's Report on Health Promotion and Disease Prevention noted:

> Physical fitness activities affect health in many ways.
>
> People who exercise regularly report that they feel better, have more energy, often require less sleep. Regular exercisers often lose excess weight as well as improve muscular strength and flexibility. Many also experience psychologic benefits including enhanced self-esteem, greater self-reliance, decreased anxiety, and relief from mild depression.
>
> Moreover, many adopt a more healthy lifestyle—abandoning smoking, excessive drinking, and poor nutritional habits.
>
> Sustained exercise improves the efficiency of the heart and increases the amount of oxygen the body can process in a given period of time. Compared to non-exercisers, people who engage in regular physical activity have been observed to have one and a half to two times lower risk of developing cardiovascular disease, and even lower risk of sudden death.

Two Misconceptions

Two mistaken ideas about exercise and weight control are still widely prevalent. One is that it takes great amounts of

---

Regular physical activity is important for maintaining health and preventing many diseases.

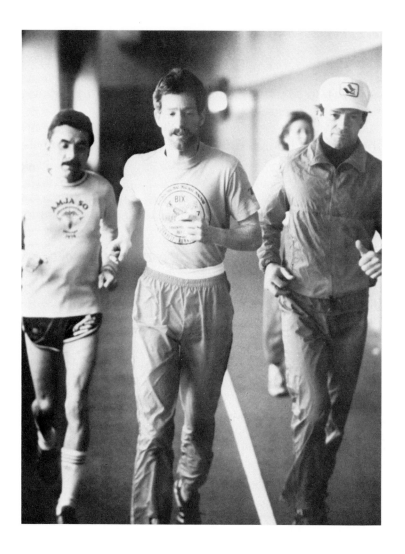

time and effort to use up enough calories to have any significant effect on weight. The other is that exercise is self-defeating: that it increases appetite and therefore, in the end, increases rather than decreases weight.

The time and effort misconception is based on the notion that exercise has to be done in a single uninterrupted session. To be sure, it sounds formidable that it can take 6 hours of jogging to use up 3600 calories, or about a pound of fat, but the jogging does not have to be done all at once. If

There have been dramatic demonstrations of the weight-control value of exercise.

one has to walk 35 miles to lose a pound, walking just one additional mile a day for 35 days will easily take off the pound and, if continued, cut off 10 pounds a year.

There have been dramatic demonstrations of the weight-control value of exercise. For example, in one study the daily food intake of a group of university students was doubled from 3000 to 6000 calories. At the same time, daily exercise was stepped up markedly. There was no gain in weight.

Also worth noting: Body weight affects energy expenditure whatever the activity—walking, jogging, tennis, or any other. For example, a 100-pound individual walking 3 miles an hour will burn up 50 calories in 15 minutes; a 200-pounder walking at the same rate for the same length of time will burn up 80 calories.

As for exercise and appetite, while thin persons will eat more after increased activity, the exercise will burn up the extra calories. Fat persons react differently: because they have large stores of fat to draw upon, only when they exercise to extremes do they experience an appetite increase. The difference between the responses of thin and fat persons is important.

To lose a pound of excess weight requires burning 3500 calories. If exercise is increased enough to use an extra 200 calories a day, that would add up to 73,000 calories in a year and a total loss of 20 pounds.

Moreover, some recent studies indicate that the calorie-burning effects of exercise continue beyond the exercise period. During vigorous activity, metabolic body processes speed up; afterward, they slow gradually. Thus the speeded-up use of energy continues for a time even after exercise is stopped.

ENERGY EQUIVALENTS OF FOOD CALORIES EXPRESSED IN MINUTES OF ACTIVITY

Food	Calories*	Activity†				
		Walking, min	Riding bicycle, min	Swimming, min	Running, min	Reclining, min
Apple (large)	101	19	12	9	5	78
Banana (small)	88	17	11	8	4	68
Beans, green (1 cup)	27	5	3	2	1	21
Beer (1 glass)	114	22	14	10	6	88
Bread and butter	78	15	10	7	4	60
Cake (2-layer, $\frac{1}{12}$)	356	68	43	32	18	274
Carbonated beverage (1 glass)	106	20	13	9	5	82
Carrot, raw	42	8	5	4	2	32
Cheese, cottage (1 tbsp)	27	5	3	2	1	21
Cheese, cheddar	111	21	14	10	6	85
Cookie, plain (0.11 oz)	15	3	2	1	1	12
Cookie, chocolate chip	51	10	6	5	3	39
Doughnut	151	29	18	13	8	116
Egg, fried	110	21	13	10	6	85
Egg, boiled	77	15	9	7	4	59
French dressing (1 tbsp)	59	11	7	5	3	45
Ice cream ($\frac{1}{6}$ qt)	193	37	24	17	10	148
Ice cream soda	255	49	31	23	13	196
Ice milk ($\frac{1}{6}$ qt)	144	28	18	13	7	111
Gelatin, with cream	117	23	14	10	6	90
Malted milk shake	502	97	61	45	26	386
Mayonnaise (1 tbsp)	92	18	11	8	5	71
Milk (1 glass)	166	32	20	15	9	128
Milk, skim (1 glass)	81	16	10	7	4	62
Milk shake	421	81	51	38	22	324
Orange (medium)	68	13	8	6	4	52
Orange juice (1 glass)	120	23	15	11	6	92
Pancake with syrup	124	24	15	11	6	95
Peach (medium)	46	9	6	4	2	35
Peas, green ($\frac{1}{2}$ cup)	56	11	7	5	3	43
Pie, apple ($\frac{1}{6}$)	377	73	46	34	19	290
Pie, raisin ($\frac{1}{6}$)	437	84	53	39	23	336
Pizza, cheese ($\frac{1}{8}$)	180	35	22	16	9	138
Potato chips (1 serving)	108	21	13	10	6	83
Sherbert ($\frac{1}{6}$ qt)	177	34	22	16	9	136
Spaghetti (1 serving)	396	76	48	35	20	305
Strawberry shortcake	400	77	49	36	21	308

* *Calorie* is used here as it is commonly used in discussions of nutrition; each "calorie" is actually equivalent to 1000 calories, or 1 kilocalorie (kcal).

† The energy cost of walking for a 154-lb individual is 5.2 Cal/min at 3.5 mi/h; riding a bicycle is 8.2 Cal/min; swimming, 11.2 Cal/min; running, 19.4 Cal/min and reclining, 1.3 Cal/min.

SOURCE: G. A. Levey, *Vegetarian Times*, 6:28, 1980, adapted from Frank Konishi, "Food Energy Equivalents of Various Activities," *Journal of the American Dietetic Association*, Vol. 46: 186, 1965.

AVERAGE ENERGY EXPENDITURE DURING RECREATIONAL ACTIVITIES

Light exercise (4 Cal/min)	Moderate exercise (7 Cal/min)	Heavy exercise (10 Cal/min)
Dancing (slow step)	Badminton (singles)	Calisthenics (vigorous)
Gardening (light)	Cycling (9.5 mi/h)	Climbing stairs (up and down)
Golf	Dancing (fast step)	Cycling (12 mi/h)
Table tennis	Gardening (heavy)	Handball, squash, paddleball
Volleyball	Stationary cycling (moderately fast)	Jogging
Walking (3 mi/h)	Swimming (30 yd/min)	Skipping rope
	Tennis (singles)	Stationary cycling (fast)
	Walking (4.5 mi/h)	Stationary jogging
		Swimming (40 yd/min)

A Calorie-Control Menu

Your Diet—What Is Sensible for You?

It may be that by continuing to eat everything you now eat but with a little moderation—a cutback here and there—you can lost weight. There is no need to rush. It took a long time for you to become overweight. You should expect it to take a reasonable time for your weight to drop down to the desired level.

It makes no sense to try to give up, all at once, all the foods you love. You are likely to feel tortured and unlikely to stick for long with such deprivation. As long as you are already eating a balanced and varied diet, it makes sense just to eat a bit less of most of the things you are eating now.

Or you may do best with a daily meal plan. If so, you will find that the guidelines we have used successfully at Executive Health Examiners may work for you.

An Essential Variety

When "Nutrition and Your Health: Dietary Guidelines for Americans" was issued recently by two government de-

CALORIE-CONTROL MENU

Meal	Day						
	1	2	3	4	5	6	7
Breakfast	Banana slices Popover 1 slice of cheese	2 chopped dates in oatmeal with cinnamon and skim milk	Sliced mango Canadian bacon in orange sauce Whole wheat toast	Fresh-fruit-and-yogurt shake	Cantaloupe with cottage cheese 1 slice of banana bread	Fruit compote with French toast	Melon balls Egg baked in tomato shell
Lunch	Tomato stuffed with chicken salad Whole wheat roll	Salad niçoise Pumpernickel roll	Flavored farmer's cheese on bed of watercress salad Comice pear sections	Insalata di frutti di mare (seafood salad) Sourdough roll	Roast chicken on pumpernickel raisin bread	Oriental scallops over rice Poached peach	Grapefruit frappe Bagel with smoked whitefish
Dinner	Honeydew melon with Nova Scotia zuppa di pesce (fish soup) Arrugula salad Baked apple	Tarragon chicken and vegetables Hearts of palm salad Apricot fluff	Egg flower soup Oriental beef with pea pods over rice Strawberries au kirsch	Vegetarian stuffed eggplant Spinach and mandarin orange salad Applesauce froth	Artichoke vinaigrette Filets of perch sage Herbed baked tomato Brandied pears	Brussel sprouts with caviar Veal chop baked in vermouth Baked acorn squash Raspberry yogurt parfait	Chicken and asparagus with salsa verde Parsleyed potatoes Gingered papaya with lime

partments—the Department of Agriculture and the Department of Health and Human Services—it listed as the very first guideline: Eat a variety of foods.

It is a concise, vital statement—very worthwhile excerpting here:

> You need about 40 different nutrients to stay healthy. These include vitamins and minerals, as well as amino acids (from proteins), essential fatty acids (from vegetable oils and animal fats), and sources of energy (calories from carbohydrates, proteins, and fats). These nutrients are in the foods you normally eat.
>
> Most foods contain more than one nutrient. Milk, for example, provides proteins, fats, sugars, riboflavin and other B-vitamins, vitamin A, calcium, and phosphorus—among other nutrients.
>
> No single food item supplies all the essential nutrients in the amounts that you need. Milk, for instance, contains very little iron or vitamin C. You should, therefore, eat a variety of foods to assure an adequate diet.
>
> The greater the variety, the less likely you are to develop either a deficiency or an excess of any single nutrient. Variety also reduces your likelihood of being exposed to excessive amounts of contaminants in any single food item.
>
> One way to assure variety and, with it, a well-balanced diet is to select foods each day from each of several major groups: for example, fruits and vegetables; cereals, breads, and grains; meat, poultry, eggs, and fish; dry peas and beans, such as soybeans, kidney beans, lima beans, and black-eyed peas, which are good vegetable sources of protein; and milk, cheese, and yogurt.
>
> Fruits and vegetables are excellent sources of vitamins, especially vitamins C and A. Whole grain and enriched breads, cereals, and grain products provide B-vitamins, iron, and energy. Meats supply protein, fat, iron and other minerals, as well as several vitamins, including thiamine and vitamin B_{12}. Dairy products are major sources of calcium and other nutrients.
>
> TO ASSURE YOURSELF AN ADEQUATE DIET, eat a variety of foods daily, including selections of fruits; vegetables; whole grains and enriched breads, cereals, and grain products; milk, cheese, and yogurt; meats, poultry, fish, and eggs; and legumes (dry peas and beans).

Cutback Maneuvers

Now, assuming you are getting variety, consider what moderation can do.

Look at the cutbacks in eating habits for examples of what individual small omissions can accomplish in terms of weight loss over a period of 1 year. Would several of these be enough to accomplish your weight-loss goal?

Remember that slow loss is not really a luxury. It gives you a chance to lose fat, not just muscle tissue or body fluids —and to form new, better eating habits.

CUTBACKS: CHANGE YOUR EATING HABITS JUST A LITTLE BIT

Food	If you omit	How often	Loss per year
Butter or margarine	1 pat	Daily	3½ lb
Bread or toast	1 slice	Daily	6 lb
Scrambled egg	1	Once a week	1½ lb
Medium-fried bacon	2 slices	Once a week	1½ lb
Pork and beans	½ serving	Once a week	2½ lb
Rice	½ serving	Once a week	1 lb
Bread stuffing	½ serving	Once a week	1 lb
Baking powder biscuit	1	Once a week	2 lb
Creamed cottage cheese	1 cup	Once a week	3 lb
Yogurt (plain)	1 cup	Once a week	2 lb
Avocado	½	Once a week	2½ lb
Oil and vinegar salad dressing	1 tbsp instead of 2	Twice a week	1½ lb
Whole roasted peanuts	¼ cup	Once a week	3 lb
Potato chips	10 medium	Once a week	1½ lb
Crackers	2 instead of 4	Twice a week	1 lb
Most cheese	1 oz	Once a week	1½ lb
Wine	3 oz	Once a week	1 lb
Beer	12-oz can	Once a week	2½ lb
Carbonated drinks	8-oz glass	Once a week	1 lb
Ice cream soda	1	Once a week	5 lb
Chocolate cake with chocolate frosting	1 slice	Once a week	4 lb
Sugar	1 tsp	Daily	1½ lb
Doughnut	1	Once a week	2 lb
Pie	½ slice	Twice a week	3½ lb
Jam or jelly	1 tbsp	Twice a week	1½ lb

THE EXECUTIVE CALORIE COUNTDOWN GUIDE

High-calorie choice*	Lower-calorie substitution*	Calories saved
APPETIZERS AND SNACKS		
1 cup New England clam chowder (275)	1 cup Manhattan clam chowder (100)	175
1 cup split pea soup (200)	1 cup consommé (25)	175
6 fried oysters (250)	6 raw oysters (80)	170
1 oz Swiss or American cheese (105)	1 oz farmer's cheese, plain (70)	35
1 tbsp cream cheese (53)	1 tbsp cottage cheese (18)	35
10 thin wheat crackers (90)	10 oyster crackers (30)	60
10 mixed nuts (94)	10 pretzels, very thin sticks (10)	84
10 potato chips (108)	10 cheese tidbits (20)	88
5 Triscuit or Ritz crackers (100)	5 pieces raw carrots or cauliflower (15)	85
2 tbsp roasted peanuts (172)	2 tbsp raisins (58)	114
1 cup buttered popcorn (172)	1 cup plain popcorn (82)	90
BEVERAGES		
1 cup whole milk, 3.5% fat (160)	1 cup skim milk or buttermilk (85)	75
1 gin and tonic, 8 oz (185)	1 wine spritzer, 2 oz wine (49)	136
1 Manhattan or martini (160)	$3\frac{1}{2}$ oz dry wine (85)	75
12 oz beer (150)	12 oz light beer (95)	55
8 oz cola, tonic water, or bitter lemon (100)	8 oz club soda (2)	98
$\frac{1}{2}$ cup grape juice (75)	$\frac{1}{2}$ cup tomato juice (25)	50
MEAT, FISH, POULTRY, EGGS		
3 oz grilled hamburger on bun (400)	3 oz roast beef on roll (300)	100
6 oz Swiss steak (630)	6 oz veal cutlet in wine (235)	395
$\frac{1}{2}$ fried chicken (464)	6 oz broiled chicken (257)	207
5 oz breaded fried perch (320)	5 oz broiled fish (240)	80
6 oz fried shrimp (380)	6 oz boiled shrimp (200)	180
1 fried egg (120)	1 poached or boiled egg (85)	35
2 strips bacon, crisp (96)	1 slice Canadian bacon (65)	31
BREADS AND STARCHES		
1 slice bread or toast (60)	2 pieces melba toast on Rykrisp (40)	20
1 Danish pastry (250)	1 plain roll (110)	140
1 cup granola-type cereal (500)	1 cup corn flakes (95)	405
$\frac{1}{2}$ cup fried rice (175)	$\frac{1}{2}$ cup rice, plain (70)	105
$\frac{1}{2}$ cup lasagna (175)	$\frac{1}{2}$ cup noodles, plain (95)	80
VEGETABLES		
20 french fries (270)	1 medium baked potato, plain (90)	180
$\frac{1}{2}$ cup potato salad (125)	$\frac{1}{2}$ cup vegetable salad, raw, no dressing (20)	105
$\frac{1}{2}$ cup cole slaw (65)	$\frac{1}{2}$ cup shredded raw cabbage (15)	50

THE EXECUTIVE
CALORIE COUNTDOWN GUIDE (Continued)

High-calorie choice*	Lower-calorie substitution*	Calories saved
½ cup corn kernels (70)	½ cup green beans, cooked (14)	56
½ cup candied sweet potatoes (150)	½ cup winter squash, mashed (50)	100
DESSERTS AND SWEETS		
Apple pie, ⅙ of 9-in pie (410)	1 baked apple, sweetened (160)	250
½ cup apple brown betty (211)	1 medium apple (88)	123
1 piece chocolate cake with icing (400)	1 piece angel cake (121)	279
2 chocolate chip cookies (104)	3 vanilla wafers (51)	53
¾ cup bread pudding with raisins (314)	½ cup gelatin, plain (81)	233
½ cup vanilla ice cream (145)	½ cup orange ice (72)	73
½ cup chocolate ice cream (150)	½ cup chocolate ice milk (102)	48
1 chocolate ice cream bar (144)	1 twin popsicle bar (95)	49
1 caramel candy (42)	1 hard candy, butterscotch (21)	21
½ oz chocolate mints (67)	1 chocolate kiss (21)	46
SAUCES AND COOKING INGREDIENTS		
2 tbsp meat gravy (82)	2 tbsp soy sauce (16)	66
½ cup sour cream (227)	½ cup yogurt, low-fat (65)	162
¼ cup heavy cream (211)	¼ cup evaporated milk (70)	141
1 tbsp butter (100)	Spray-type oil (PAM) (2 seconds) (8)	92
1 tbsp mayonnaise (101)	1 tbsp mayonnaise-type dressing (Miracle Whip) (61)	40
1 tbsp olive oil (124)	1 tbsp vinegar (2)	122

* Numbers in parentheses are "calories," or "large calories," as meant in common discussions of nutrition; each "calorie" is actually equivalent to 1 kilocalorie (kcal), or 1000 calories.
SOURCE: Riska Platt, M.S., R.D.

If cutback maneuvers are not likely to be enough, you might want to try substitution maneuvers.

Substitution Maneuvers

In many cases, the caloric content of similar foods varies greatly despite the fact that the looks, tastes, and satisfactions may be quite similar. So substitutions often can be made readily and can prove quite satisfying, while saving many calories and contributing markedly to weight control.

At Executive Health Examiners, we have found "The Executive Calorie Countdown Guide" to be helpful for many executives.

Executive Health Examiners Weight-Control Plans

Many of our executive clients find it helpful to use a definite weight-control food plan—a balanced weight reduction diet simplified by the use of "exchange lists."

As you see in the exchange lists, there are six lists: breads, grains, and starchy vegetables; meat, fish, eggs, and cheese; skim milk; vegetables; fruits; and fats. Foods in the lists are grouped according to their nutrient similarities.

In the amounts shown, all the foods in one list are equal in value to each other. The average caloric value for all foods in a list is indicated at the top of the list.

The term *exchange* denotes that you can exchange a serving of one food within a list for a serving of another food within the same list. For example, in list 5, fruits, you can exchange $\frac{1}{3}$ cup of apple juice for $\frac{1}{2}$ cup of orange juice, if you prefer the latter, or either for half a cantaloupe.

However, a food in one list cannot be traded for a food in another unless so indicated.

Note, too, that *to plan a diet lower in cholesterol and saturated fat, you must avoid or eat less of those foods which appear in italics, using others in the same lists instead.*

How to Use Your Plan

Since 1 pound of body fat represents 3500 calories, a reduction in intake of 500 calories a day should lead to a weight loss of about 1 pound a week.

The Recommended Daily Allowance (RDA) of calories for adults aged 23 to 50 is 2000 for women and 2700 for men. Despite differences in physical activity and body build, most adults can lose weight successfully on a caloric intake ranging from 1200 to 1800 calories.

The following table shows you the total number of daily exchanges or servings for each of three calorie levels: 1200,

EXCHANGE LISTS

List 1: breads, grains, and starchy vegetables* (Average: 68 Cal)		List 2: meat, fish, eggs, and cheese (Average: 73 Cal)		List 3: skim milk‡ (Average: 100 Cal)	
BREAD PRODUCTS		**LOWER FAT**		**NONFAT MILK, FORTIFIED**	
Bread (all types)	1 slice	Veal	1 oz	Milk, skim	1 cup
Bagel (small)	½	Poultry (no skin)	1 oz†	Milk, evaporated, skim	1 cup
Bun (hamburger or		Fish:		Milk, powdered, skim	½ cup
frankfurter)	½	Any fresh or frozen	1 oz	Buttermilk, skim	1 cup
English muffin	½	Canned:		Yogurt (plain, unflavored),	
Roll (plain, small)	1	Salmon, tuna, mackerel,		made with skim milk	1 cup
CRACKERS		crab, or lobster	¼ cup	**LOW-FAT MILK, FORTIFIED**	
Saltines (squares)	6	Clams, oysters, or		99% fat free	1 cup
Melba toast	3	scallops	5 oz		
Matzoh	½	*Shrimp*	1 oz		
CEREAL		Sardines (drained)	3		
Dry, unsweetened	¾ cup	Cottage cheese (2% fat)	¼ cup		
Cooked	½ cup	Cheese (less than 5% fat)	1 oz		
GRAINS		**HIGHER FAT**			
Rice (cooked)	½ cup	*Beef:* steak, roast, or ground	1 oz		
Spaghetti, noodles, or		*Lamb* (lean)	1 oz		
macaroni (cooked)	½ cup	*Pork* or *ham* (lean)	1 oz		
Flour	2½ tsp	*Liver* or *organ meats*	1 oz		
STARCHY VEGETABLES		Cheese:			
Corn	⅓ dup	Hard types	1 oz		
Corn on cob (small)	1	Parmesan	3 tbsp		
Baked beans (no pork)	¼ cup	Mozzarella or farmer's	1 oz		
Dried peas or beans		Peanut butter	2 tbsp		
(cooked)	½ cup	*Frankfurter*	½		
Peas (frozen, canned)	½ cup	*Eggs*	1		
Potatoes, white					
(baked or boiled, small)	1				
Yams, sweet	¼ cup				
Winter squash	½ cup				
OTHER					
Ice cream (*plain*)					
(omit 1 fat exchange)	⅓ cup				

* Broth-based soup: 1 cup = 1 bread + 1 fat.   † ¼ chicken = 3 oz.   ‡ If *whole milk* is used, omit 2 fat exchanges.

SOURCE: Riska Platt, M.S., R.D.

List 4: vegetables (Average: 25 Cal)		List 5: fruits§ (Average: 70 Cal)		List 6: fats (Average: 45 Cal)	
One exchange is ½ cup:		Apple	1 small	*Butter*	1 tsp
Beets		Apple juice	⅓ cup	Margarine	1 tsp
Carrots		Applesauce	½ cup	*Bacon, crisp*	1 strip
Onions		(unsweetened)		*Cream, light*	2 tbsp
Rhubarb		Apricots, fresh	2 medium	*Cream, sour*	2 tbsp
Rutabaga		Apricots, dried	4 halves	*Cream, heavy*	1 tbsp
Sauerkraut		Banana	½ small	*Cream cheese*	1 tbsp
Tomatoes		Berries, all kinds	½ cup	French dressing	1 tbsp
Tomato juice		Cherries	10 large	Italian dressing	1 tbsp
Turnips		Cider	⅓ cup	Mayonnaise	1 tbsp
The following raw vegetables may		Dates	2	Salad dressing	
be used as desired. If cooked,		Figs, fresh	1	(mayonnaise type)	2 tbsp
½ cup only:		Figs, dried	1	Oil	1 tbsp
Asparagus		Grapefruit	1	Olives	5 small
Beans, green or wax		Grapefruit juice	½ cup	Nuts	6 small
Broccoli		Grapes	12	*Pork sausage*	½ link
Brussels sprouts		Grape juice	¼ cup	Avocado (4-in diameter)	⅛
Cabbage		Mango	½ small		
Cauliflower		Melons:			
Celery		Canteloupe	½ small		
Cucumbers		Honeydew	⅛ medium		
Eggplant		Watermelon	1 cup		
Escarole		Nectarine	1 small		
Greens: all kinds		Orange	1 small		
Lettuce: all kinds		Orange juice	½ cup		
Mushrooms		Papaya	¾ cup		
Okra		Peach	1 medium		
Parsley		Pear	1 small		
Peppers: green or red		Pineapple	½ cup		
Radishes		Pineapple juice	⅓ cup		
Spinach		Plums	2 medium		
Squash, summer or zucchini		Prunes	2 medium		
Watercress		Prune juice	¼ cup		
		Raisins	2 tbsp		
		Tangerine	1 medium		

§ Fresh or canned without sugar.

NUMBER OF EXCHANGES (SERVINGS) ALLOWED FOR VARIOUS CALORIE LEVELS

List	1200 Cal Plan A	1200 Cal Plan B	1500 Cal Plan A	1500 Cal Plan B	1800 Cal Plan A	1800 Cal Plan B
1 Starch group	2	4	3	6	4	8
2 Meat group	8	6	10	7	13	7
3 Milk group	1	2	1	2	1	2
4 Vegetable group	3	2	3	2	5	3
5 Fruit group	3	2	3	3	3	4
6 Fat group	2	2	4	3	3	4

1500, and 1800. For each level, two plans are provided; you may choose either or switch between them at will.

Special Notes About Your Plan

Free Foods You may have unlimited amounts of the following: coffee or tea (but remember to count added dairy products and sweetener); bouillon, broth, or consommé (without fat); unsweetened gelatin; unsweetened pickles; and carbonated or soda water (without sugar).

Low-Calorie Additions You may have moderate amounts of the following: baking soda or baking powder; celery seed or celery salt; chili powder; flavoring extracts (e.g., vanilla); garlic; herbs (curry, sage, thyme, etc.); horseradish; lemon or lime juice; mint; mustard; onion; pepper; paprika; salt; spices (cinnamon, ginger, etc.); vinegar; dry wine for cooking; and diet sodas, low-calorie beverages, or low-calorie salad dressings (among them, not to exceed a total of 25 calories daily).

Avoid Cake, candy, chewing gum, cookies, honey, jam and jelly, pastries, soft drinks, sugar, syrup, and tonic water.

Cooking Methods Broil, bake, steam, or boil your foods. Trim fat from meat before cooking. Any fats used in cooking must be counted. Adding dry wine and herbs will enhance the flavor of foods cooked without oils.

Food Labels   A label indicating "dietetic" food does not mean the food can be eaten in unlimited amounts.

A good diet is one that:

- Is nutritionally sound—which means that it provides all the necessary nutrients and therefore contains a wide variety of foods. The aim of a reducing diet is to help decrease body fat without damaging body structure.
- With some additions can become a basic pattern of eating for the rest of your life.
- Consists of foods that are appetizing and pleasant to eat.
- Helps train the appetite and encourages you to develop a pattern of eating at regular intervals.
- Provides food with staying power—the power to satisfy your appetite and prevent excessive hunger.
- Is built around a nucleus of familiar foods. It should be adaptable to your living situation.
- Can be matched to the individual. Different people lose weight at different calorie levels, and diets should be planned accordingly.

A bad diet is one that:

- Has a limited choice of food—which leads to feelings of deprivation and monotony and does not provide all necessary nutrients.
- Requires special foods that make it difficult to follow in most living situations.
- Leads to rapid weight loss, which may be detrimental to your health.
- Does not establish a pattern to follow for life.

Riska Platt, M.S., R.D., EHE nutrition consultant

DO YOU KNOW GOOD FROM BAD WHEN IT COMES TO DIETS?

A label indicating "dietetic" food does not mean the food can be eaten in unlimited amounts.

HAVE A SPRITZER

Something I suggest to executives who want to cut down their drinking at parties is that they have a wine or vermouth spritzer in a large glass. If they sip it slowly, it will last much longer and people won't come around to refill their glass so often.

With scotch and water, the first half glass tastes awful; the next is much better. The next six —terrific—but they're consuming all those calories.

An EHE physician

When You Dine Out

It is often said that executive business lunches and other restaurant meals make weight control impossible.

That is not true.

Many weight-conscious executives are very successful dieters. It is not uncommon to find executives who eat ten or more meals weekly at restaurants and still manage to control their weight.

Most of them are assertive. They make special requests, and if the requests are not strictly honored, they find other restaurants that are happy to comply with them. Finding such restaurants is becoming easier and easier as patrons are becoming more and more demanding about good nutrition.

There is no reason to have any hesitation about specifying how you want your food prepared—baked, broiled or steamed, for example, instead of fried and with sauces and salad dressings served on the side.

In addition to avoiding such high-calorie extras, as sauces, crackers, rolls, sour cream, butter, and dressings, weight-conscious executives often leave unfinished a significant part of oversized portions. They make menu selections carefully. When being host or hosted at even the finest steak and chop house, for example, they may order broiled fish, spinach salad without bacon bits, and white wine and have a fine meal, free of excessive calories.

Weight-conscious individuals should choose beverages carefully too. Many have conceded that martinis and other alcoholic beverages contribute nothing but calories to the meal and therefore have switched to club soda or to one of

It is often said that executive business lunches and other restaurant meals make weight control impossible.

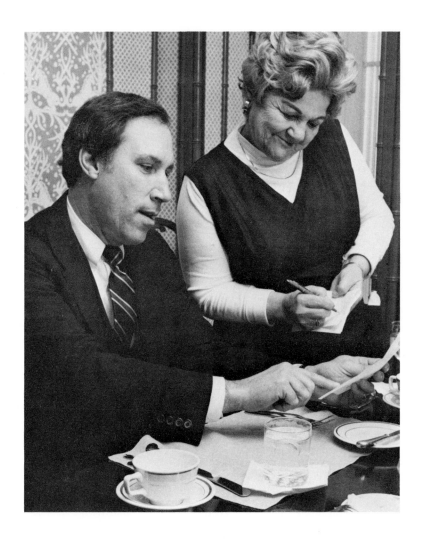

the mineral waters that are currently popular. Others have cut calories by drinking wine spritzers, which contain only an ounce or two of wine with calorie-free soda water.

Q: What do I tell a 20-pound overweight executive who tells me, "I'm forever dieting," "I can't lose weight," "It's not easy," "I'm on the road all the time"?

A: I say: "No red meats because of the high fat content. The better the red meat, the more the fat content."

He says: "I cut the fat off."

"That's not the part that tastes good. It's the nice marbling that tastes good."

I say: "Order fish or chicken, broiled or baked. They're low-fat, low-cholesterol foods with good nutrients. No fried foods, including french fries. And play down the alcohol. It's calorie-loaded, a good fuel—that's why they put it in gas tanks."

And I tell him: "Have a giant salad before eating. No more than 1 tablespoon of oil. Toss the lettuce a long time; the exercise is good for you. And I mean a giant salad—like half a head of lettuce, a whole tomato, a whole cucumber, scallions—plenty of food."

And I say: "You want a chocolate mousse at a restaurant where its absolutely delicious? Sure, have it on occasion—but then don't sit watching football on television with 2 pounds of candy. Save it for the mousse."

I say, too: "Once you're at your right weight, maybe you can add red meat once or twice a week and hold it steady."

Does it work? I've had many, many patients come back for their next checkup and they've lost 20 pounds—some even 30—over the year. It works because they thought it was a sensible plan—no calorie counting."

An EHE physician

THE EXECUTIVE LUNCH

High-calorie meal	Calories	Calorie-conscious meal	Calories
$3\frac{1}{2}$ oz martini	160	Wine spritzer (2 oz wine mixed with club soda)	50
1 cup French onion soup au gratin	275	1 cup consommé	25
16 oz broiled prime steak	1100	16 oz flounder, broiled with wine or lemon juice	310
$\frac{1}{2}$ cup hashed brown potatoes	225	Baked potato with 1 pat butter	125
Tossed salad with 1 tbsp Italian dressing	100	Tossed salad with 1 tbsp vinegar	25
Chocolate eclair	275	1 cup berries	100
Coffee with 1 tbsp cream	30	Black coffee	0
Total	2165	Total	635

SOURCE: Riska Platt, M.S., R.D.

When You Travel

Travel can make weight control more difficult, but many executives have learned to cope effectively by using some of the following techniques:

* Plan ahead. *Most executives have an agenda which includes many scheduled meals. It is usually easy to predict the type of meal (sometimes even the actual foods) that will be served. Plan for light meals or snacks when nothing is scheduled.*

* Retain the same eating habits you have established at home, *if they are good ones. For example, do not eat a huge breakfast if you normally have only a small bowl of cereal.*

* Limit alcohol intake. *Alcoholic beverages are high in calories and do not enhance mental acuity for conducting business.*

* Exercise. *Jog, use a jump rope, or climb the hotel stairs if your physician approves. Otherwise, walk as much as possible.*

* Do not use food to compensate for being away from home; *it is not an adequate substitute anyway. Even if large and frequent meals are included with the hotel room or on the expense account, an executive who eats them all will end up paying for them in more ways than one.*

* Be assertive. *Request in advance the special meals that are readily available on airplanes and ask for substitutions at restaurants.*

Making Use of Behavior-Modification Techniques

We have found at Executive Health Examiners that changing eating habits through behavior-modification techniques is very important in successful weight reduction and weight control. We put major emphasis on it.

Commonly, eating too much is a learned behavior, a habitual response to stimuli in the social environment. Behavior modification applies the principles of psychology to changing the habits that make for overeating.

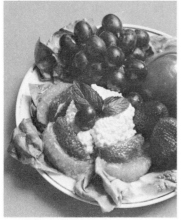

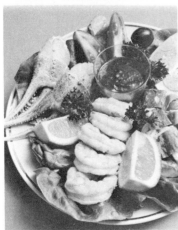

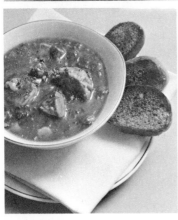

All of us sometimes eat without being hungry. It appears that the overweight, however, eat in large measure because of environmental cues—time of day, odors, palatability of food, or sight of food. They often nibble without thinking about it, while watching television or reading.

The First Step

Take an inventory of your eating habits. Keep an eating diary of everything you eat each day, noting:

* *the type and amount of food*

* *where and when the food is eaten*

* *the time spent eating*

* *any activity while eating*

* *people you eat with*

* *your mood when you eat—how you feel at the time*

* *any events precipitating the eating*

* *how hungry (or not hungry) you are when you eat*

A bore and a bother? It may well be at the very start, but you are likely to find that it is not only valuable but interesting as well.

For one thing, just monitoring their intake of food helps many people to cut down. You may find that you are less likely to order a rich dessert at lunch or down a handful of peanuts in the evening when you realize you are obligated to yourself to write it down.

You will also be getting, as you may never have had before, an accurate picture of those eating habits that are causing trouble.

Analyze the Record

You may be surprised at what the record tells you about yourself.

At a recent New York Medical College symposium, Sami A. Hashim, M.D., of St. Luke's Hospital Center in New York, reported on research he and his colleagues had done to show the degree to which the eating habits of obese people are controlled by influences other than their physiological needs.

Lean and obese volunteers were brought to St. Luke's, where they were fed tasteless though nutritious food served in a variety of ways.

First, the food was offered through a tube. "The obese patient reduced his intake drastically," Dr. Hashim reported, "consuming about one-tenth of the calories he needed to maintain his weight." The lean subjects, however, ate just enough to maintain their body weight.

Then the situation was changed in various ways to make eating the same food somewhat more attractive. Nothing the researchers did had any effect on the eating of the lean people, but the obese subjects altered their eating drastically.

"When we switched the automatic feeding from a tube to a paper cup," reported Dr. Hashim, "the obese patient would consume twice as much. We put the formula in a crystal goblet and he doubled his intake again. We put a candle in the room and he consumed even more."

The hopeful note: The responses to these influences are learned responses—so they can be unlearned.

In another experiment, Albert J. Stunkard, M.D., of the Hospital of the University of Pennsylvania, and other investigators found that although behavior modification does not produce as rapid a weight loss as antiappetite drug treatment or a combination of behavior modification and drug therapy, it produced better maintenance of weight loss.

The three types of treatment were compared in 134 obese subjects: those who received an appetite suppressant, fenfluramine, lost an average of 32 pounds over a 6-month period; those who received combined treatment lost 33.6 pounds; those on behavior modification alone lost 24 pounds.

But a 1-year follow up showed a striking reversal of results: Behavior-modification patients had regained only 4 pounds while the drug-treated patients had regained 18 pounds and the combined-treatment patients, $23\frac{1}{2}$ pounds.

Thus, as the investigators noted, behavior therapy is superior from the standpoints of better maintenance of weight loss and lower costs. Apparently, adding a drug only interferes with the long-term effects of behavior modification.

TWO NOTEWORTHY EXPERIMENTS

You may find that you eat more often or much more quickly than you thought you did or that you get a desire for food under certain circumstances—on passing the refrigerator, when you're fatigued or bored, or at some particular time of day—even though you're not hungry at all.

This behavior profile can help you to detect any eating behavior which is associated with circumstances or emotional stress rather than with hunger.

Once aware of what is going on, you will recognize, of course, that food is not a suitable response to fatigue or boredom. You can exert control when it is needed and, in the process, find more appropriate responses.

If, for example, you find from your record that you do considerable snacking when you settle down to watch television, you can find a solution for that. One obvious possibility, of course, is to watch television less.

Suggested Behavior Modifications

* *Eat slowly and enjoy your food. Many studies indicate that when you make a deliberate decision to eat and then take the time to enjoy the eating thoroughly, you will experience a greater sense of satisfaction, even though you may be consuming fewer calories.*

* *Eat slowly to give your appetite a chance to be satisfied. If you eat a meal in less than 20 minutes, you are eating too fast to enjoy it. Moreover, it takes about 20 minutes for the brain to register "Enough." Therefore if you finish a meal in less time, you are more likely to reach for seconds because you still feel hungry.*

* *Make use of as many of the following techniques as you find helpful to slow your eating:*

* *Take small bites.*

* *Chew your food longer, savoring each bite. (You will not, of course, enjoy its taste once it is "down the hatch.") In chewing use the taste buds on the right side, the left side, and then the back of the tongue before swallowing.*

* Use your napkin more often.

* Put your fork or spoon down after each bite and wait until you have swallowed before taking another forkful or spoonful of food.

* Take sips of water —or plain tea or coffee —between bites.

* Count your bites, and after every three or four, wait a minute or two before taking another.

* Pause for a few minutes in the middle of a meal.

* Concentrate on your eating. Avoid watching television or reading.

* Request your family and friends not to offer you seconds at meals or food between meals. Let them know that while offering food may commonly be equated with affection, you will regard it as far more affectionate if they don't offer you food.

Other Useful Modifications

* At home, choose one place to eat all meals and snacks.

* Sit in a chair when you eat —never stand, even for snacks.

* Use a plate and utensils —again, even for snacks.

* Even at home, avoid "family-style" eating and, instead, have food portioned on plates before it is brought to the table. Keep serving platters and bowls in the kitchen.

* At home and in restaurants, always leave at least a small amount of food on your plate.

Modified Attitudes

* Regard behavior changes as more important in the long run than immediate weight changes.

* Develop a tolerance for mild hunger. Think of it as a positive feeling.

* *Make deliberate decisions to eat; don't eat absentmindedly.*

* *Do not immediately stop eating all of your favorite foods. All of us have "sin" foods—bread or pizza or sweets. Many people on diets forbid themselves such favorites, until their craving for them finally gets out of control and they binge. Afterward they feel guilty, and many then stop dieting.*

* *Plan in advance to indulge yourself occasionally—and to make up for it by eating less of something else.*

Underweight

If you are markedly underweight or are losing weight, medical advice is important.

A chronic underweight condition or sudden loss of weight can be an indication of a health problem. It may signal the presence or onset of disease, for example, diabetes, thyroid gland overactivity (hyperthyroidism), or chronic infection.

Finding the cause and correcting it are the job of a physician.

Determining if You Are Underweight

Quite possibly, you will need the help of a physician to determine whether you are really underweight.

It is likely, of course, that you are if you are 10 to 15 pounds or more below the figures in the table on desirable weights and if, in addition, bones stick out all over your body, or your muscles do not provide adequate resilient protection to your back, thighs, and buttocks, or your face is thin and drawn.

The weight figures in the table alone may not be enough to indicate underweight. You could be the long, lean type whose weight normally falls below those figures.

Your physician, after a physical examination, including observations of the size and bony framework of your body, can determine fairly accurately whether you are under-weight. Some people worry needlessly over an underweight condition that does not actually exist, because of a "diagnosis" by well-meaning friends or relatives.

What to Do about It

If extreme thinness is not the result of an underlying medical problem, it is very likely due to not eating enough of the right kinds of food. Your physician undoubtedly will have suggestions, including some for a change in diet.

How you eat can also be important. It takes time to eat proper meals and enjoy them. A 5- or 10-minute mealtime is hardly conducive to eating more without feeling stuffed. Longer and more relaxed mealtimes may help solve your problem.

Relaxing *before* meals can be helpful too. It is difficult to eat adequately when you are either all steamed up or tired.

You may find that large portions discourage you from eating—or, on the other hand, you may have difficulty taking seconds and do better with large servings. It could be helpful, if you don't know, to determine which type you are and to determine, too, whether you eat more at family-style meals, or when food is served in predetermined portions.

Eating More

If you now eat relatively little, that can be a matter of habit—and habits can be changed. By taking an extra slice of bread or a second helping—even quite a small one—you may begin to change your eating patterns.

High-Calorie Foods

Certain vegetables—among them peas, lima beans, and po-tatoes—are higher in calories than others, particularly leafy vegetables. Try to increase your intake of higher-calorie foods, but continue to eat salads as well.

If your physician finds you have no blood-fat problems,

you may find it helpful to increase your intake of such high-calorie foods as chowders, cream soups, mayonnaise, sauces, and rich desserts.

Snacking

Snacks can add weight, and you should look for some that you will enjoy.

You may find that some—such as candy, cake, and ice cream—tend to satiate you, dulling your mealtime hunger, but there are others you can try. Peanut butter and fruit, for example, are valuable for supplying essential nutrients as well as extra calories.

Smoking

Particularly when excessive, smoking can dull the appetite and the taste buds as well. You might try cutting down. At the least, try to avoid smoking just before and during meals.

Alcohol

For some people, sipping an aperitif, such as a glass of sherry, before dinner helps stimulate their appetite. For others, a leisurely cocktail or highball is helpful. Obviously, however, alcohol should not be substituted for food.

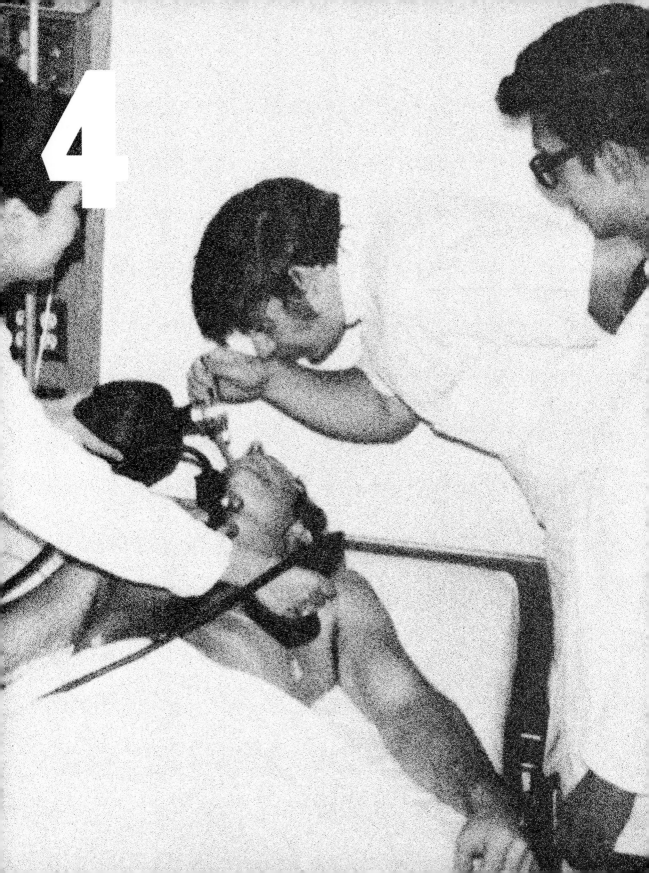

NUTRITION AND CARDIOVASCULAR DISEASE

More than two Americans each minute—some 3400 a day—suffer heart attacks. Another 1600 a day are stroke victims. Cardiovascular disease—disease of the heart and blood vessels—accounts for almost 1 million deaths a year, about 52 percent of the total.

To what extent does how we eat influence cardiovascular disease?

As you know, many risk factors have been identified, including a family history of heart attack, stroke, or sudden premature death (before age 65), a sedentary lifestyle, cigarette smoking, stress, and personality type. Other major risk factors include obesity, high blood pressure, and elevated blood cholesterol. Nutrition has a significant impact as well, because it influences all three of the latter.

We looked at obesity and how it can be attacked in Chapter 3. Now we will examine the significant nutritional aspects of blood pressure and cholesterol levels.

High Blood Pressure

Hypertension, "the silent disease," is almost incredibly common and, when neglected, extremely dangerous. It too often is neglected because it commonly remains undetected until severe damage occurs, producing such complications as stroke, heart attack, or kidney failure.

99

In the United States, 25 million people have blood pressure above 140/90 but below 160/95—"borderline hypertension"—who could help themselves by following weight-loss or weight-maintenance and salt-control programs. Another 35 million people have blood pressure of 160/95 or higher and need additional medical intervention.

Blood Pressure: What It Is and How It Is Measured

Blood pressure is simply the force exerted against the walls of arteries as blood flows through them. The pressure is produced primarily by the pumping action of the heart. It is essential for pushing the body's 5 quarts of blood through its more than 60,000 miles of blood vessels in order to get blood-transported oxygen and nutrients to all tissues in the body.

Despite earlier more primitive experiments, it was not until 1828 that a French medical student, Jean Leonard-Marie Poiseuille, thought of connecting a mercury-filled tube to an artery and measurement of blood pressure became feasible.

Almost another 70 years had to go by before an Italian physician reported a measuring instrument, the sphygmomanometer, which, like modern instruments, had a rubber cuff that could be pumped up to cut off the pulse. In 1905, a Russian physician reported a method of picking up pulse sounds by using a stethoscope, and finally, about the time of World War I, blood pressure measurements began to be taken much as they are today.

How It Works You probably made use of the principle behind the sphygmomanometer in your high-school-laboratory days. When you poured mercury into one end of a U-shaped glass tube, you promptly had two columns of mercury, one in each arm of the tube, with both columns at the same height, the weight of the mercury in one arm balancing the weight in the other.

But if you then attached a rubber bulb and short length of rubber or plastic tubing to one arm of the glass tube and squeezed the bulb, you could see that air pressure lowered the mercury level in that arm and raised it in the other.

Working in much the same way, the sphygmomanometer consists of a column of mercury, a cloth bag that is wrapped around the arm just above the elbow, and a rubber bulb. Pumping the bulb makes the cloth bag swell with air and squeeze against the underlying artery in the arm. As air pressure in the bag increases, the flow of blood through the artery is diminished and finally stopped altogether. At the same time, the level of the mercury rises because of the increase in air pressure.

Now, when the cone-shaped end of the stethoscope is placed just below the cloth bag on the artery, nothing is

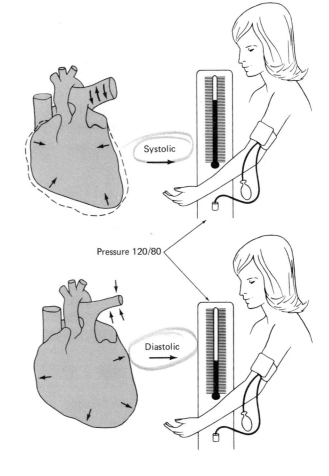

Systolic

Pressure 120/80

Diastolic

When the blood volume is increased, the heart has to pump more blood, and since the greater volume of blood is forced into a vessel of relatively fixed size, the blood pressure increases. Similarly, when the blood volume is decreased, the pressure in the artery is lowered. (From J. D. Margie & J. C. Hunt, Living with High Blood Pressure, The Hypertensive Diet Cookbook, JLS Press, Bloomfield, N.J., 1978.)

heard, because no blood is flowing through the artery, but as air is released slowly from the bag, the mercury level in the column falls because there is less air to hold it up. As more air is released, a point is reached at which the pressure of the blood pushing against the bag is able to overcome the pressure from the bag that has been cutting off the flow. As blood gets through, beats begin to be heard through the stethoscope. The mercury level at that moment marks the *systolic* blood pressure, the pressure in the artery when a beat of the heart forces a surge of blood through the circulatory system.

As still more air is released, the sound of blood pushing through the artery becomes louder and then fades. At the fading point, the mercury level marks the *diastolic* pressure, the low level reached when the heart relaxes between beats.

Since no two people are exactly alike in anything, including heartbeat force, there is a wide range of blood pressure in healthy, normal people. A systolic pressure between 100 and 140 millimeters of mercury is considered normal, as is a diastolic pressure between 60 and 90 millimeters of mercury. When pressure goes above the upper limits of normal, hypertension has to be considered.

A striking array of facts about hypertension and life and death came from a massive inter-insurance company study published in 1959 by the Society of Actuaries. It covered 4 million lives and 102,000 deaths, and it showed that blood pressures above 140/90 are abnormal and lead to higher mortality.

For example, the study revealed that a 45-year-old man with blood pressure of 150/90—hardly an extreme elevation —could expect to live 7 fewer years than if his blood pressure were not that mildly elevated.

Generally, the higher the pressure, the greater the detrimental effect. At an elevation of 160/100, the risk of premature death can be increased as much as 250 percent.

For a man of 35 with diastolic pressure of 85 millimeters of mercury and systolic pressure elevated only slightly to 142 millimeters of mercury, the mortality rate is 150 percent above average. With a diastolic pressure of 95 millimeters of mercury and systolic pressure of 145 millimeters of mercury, the mortality rate is 225 percent above average, while a sys-

INCREASE IN MORTALITY RATE FOR INSURED MEN AND WOMEN WITH RISE IN BLOOD PRESSURE*

Systolic pressure

	138–147 mmHg		148–157 mmHg		158–167 mmHg		168–177 mmHg		178–192 mmHg	
	Men	Women	Men	Women	Men	Women	Men	Women	Men	Women
1959 Build and Blood Pressure Study	55% higher	22% higher	94% higher	40% higher	144% higher	130% higher	—	—	—	—
1979 Build and Blood Pressure Study	36% higher	22% higher	68% higher	35% higher	110% higher	67% higher	124% higher	—	132% higher	—

Diastolic pressure

	88–92 mmHg		93–97 mmHg		98–102 mmHg		103–108 mmHg	
	Men	Women	Men	Women	Men	Women	Men	Women
1959 Build and Blood Pressure Study	50% higher	22% higher	88% higher	68% higher	134% higher	118% higher	162% higher	—
1979 Build and Blood Pressure Study	38% higher	33% higher	71% higher	63% higher	104% higher	83% higher	164% higher	—

* Dashes denote too few cases for analysis.

NOTE: The 1959 Build and Blood Pressure Study reflects the mortality experience among insured lives covering the years 1935 through 1954, and the 1979 Build and Blood Pressure Study reflects provisional experience among insured lives covering the years 1954 through 1972.

SOURCE: Ad Hoc Committee of the New Build and Blood Pressure Study, Association of Life Insurance Medical Directors of America and Society of Actuaries.

tolic pressure of 152 millimeters of mercury and a diastolic pressure of 95 millimeters of mercury increase the mortality rate to 300 percent above average.

In the government's Framingham, Massachusetts study, which followed more than 5000 originally healthy people for more than 30 years, heart attacks proved to be as much as five times more common over a 14-year period in those with hypertension than in others. The risk of stroke was four times as high in those with elevated pressure.

What are the effects of hypertension?

For one thing, it can cause the heart to enlarge under the burden of having to pump harder against increased pressure. The heart can tolerate the burden for years but eventually may weaken under the strain, losing a considerable degree of its pumping efficiency. This leads to congestive heart failure.

Longstanding hypertension also causes damaging changes in the arteries. The vessel walls thicken and harden, and this may favor the deposition and accumulation of cholesterol and fat (atherosclerosis) and may diminish blood flow, leading to heart attack and stroke. The same process affecting the arteries to the kidneys may lead to kidney failure.

More and more investigators now are convinced that

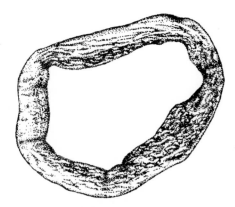

Normal Artery

The atherosclerotic process

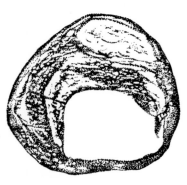

Fatty Deposits in
Vessel Wall

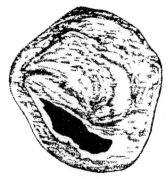

Plugged Artery with Fatty
Deposits and Clot

104   *Nutrition and Cardiovascular Disease*

Hypertension provokes atherosclerosis . . . damaging the arteries . . . but there is nothing inevitable about those and other serious consequences.

high blood pressure plays an important role in provoking atherosclerosis by increasing the stress on the linings of the arteries. There is nothing inevitable, however, about the consequences of hypertension. No matter how high the pressure, an effective antihypertension program can greatly improve life expectancy, help relieve symptoms if present, and reduce the number of complications.

It is now generally agreed also that early treatment can defer the effects of atherosclerosis and even go a long way toward preventing its development altogether.

The Kinds of Hypertension

In only about 10 percent of people with elevated blood pressure can the trouble be traced to a definite physical cause. There may be pinching, or coarctation, of a portion of the aorta, the body's main trunk-line artery emerging from the heart. Narrowing of the kidney artery can elevate pressure. So, too, can a tumor of the adrenal gland. Such abnormalities often can be corrected by surgery, and blood pressure then returns to normal.

In the remaining 90 percent of patients, the hypertension is of unknown cause and is called *essential* or *idiopathic hypertension*. Essential hypertension can be treated effectively with antihypertensive drugs, but medication may not always be required. Evidence has been growing that overweight and excessive sodium (salt) intake can be significant factors in many cases of hypertension, and the elimination of one or the other, or of both, may be all that is needed to bring blood pressure down to normal.

Overweight and Blood Pressure

Physicians have long had the impression that hypertension and obesity may be related. Today there is no longer any doubt that excess weight is an important contributing factor to the development of high blood pressure.

The Framingham study confirmed this impression. Framingham participants with hypertension were found more often to be obese than people with normal blood pressure. Also, the prevalence of hypertension at all ages increased with relative weight.

Other studies as well have shown that most people with essential hypertension, even adolescents, are overweight. Conversely, the overweight are more likely than normal-weight individuals to have hypertension or to develop it over a period of a few years. And people who are overweight and hypertensive are more likely to have severe hypertension than hypertensive patients of normal weight.

Significantly, too, many physicians over the years have observed the effectiveness of weight reduction as a treatment for hypertension. The Framingham experience also confirmed this observation. About 60 percent of Framingham hypertensives who were able to achieve a substantial weight loss were able to lower their blood pressure below hypertensive levels.

Further confirmation has come from a recent study in Israel, where 81 hypertensive patients who were 10 percent or more above their ideal weight were put on a weight-reduction program. Over a 2-month period, all lost at least 6.6 pounds, and the mean weight loss was 23 pounds. All but 2 of the 81 patients had a significant fall in blood pressure.

In the Israel study, not only did 75 percent of the obese hypertensive patients who were not on medication return to normal blood pressure when they lost weight, but, in addition, 61 percent of those who were hypertensive despite medication returned to normal blood pressure when they lost weight, with no change in medication.

At Executive Health Examiners we often see patients whose excess weight aggravates their hypertension. L.W., a prominent, 44-year-old banker, claimed that his 45 pounds of extra weight were directly related to his need to entertain

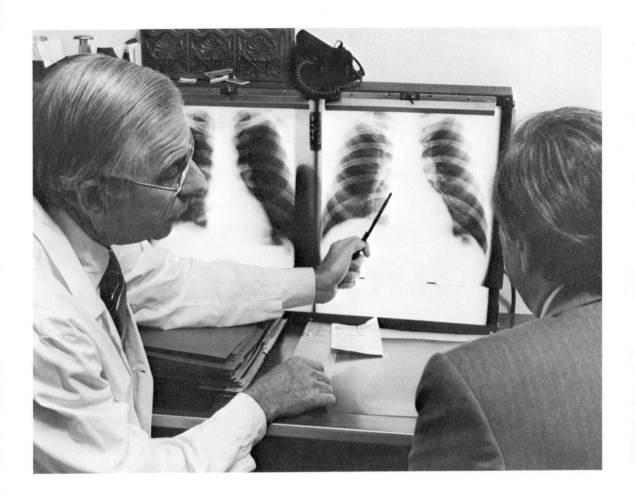

clients and personal friends at his luncheon club and popular restaurants. Recently divorced from his wife of 20 years, he spent most evenings at parties and/or restaurants.

L.W. was taking a significant amount of medication for elevated blood pressure. At Executive Health Examiners, a physician convinced him that a consultation with the nutritionist might show him how he could achieve weight loss and decrease his hypertension through diet.

That is just what happened. An individualized diet plan to cut calories and sodium intake was devised by the nutritionist. At L.W.'s request, she reviewed a collection of restaurant menus with him and discussed his dietary problems with the chef at his club. Over the next 18 months, L.W. lost

30 pounds, and the physician was able to cut the dose of hypertension medication in half. L.W. continues to work toward his goal of additional weight loss and better blood pressure control without an abrupt change in his lifestyle.

The Role of Salt

Many investigators today believe, on the basis of a sizeable body of evidence, that excessive salt intake plays a major role in hypertension, particularly when coupled with genetic predisposition to elevated blood pressure.

The late Lewis K. Dahl, M.D., of Brookhaven National Laboratory, who did a lot of the pioneering work linking salt with hypertension, first became interested in salt in 1948. At that time a rice-fruit diet was being used with some good results to treat hypertension.

What was the ingredient in the diet, Dahl wondered, that accounted for the blood pressure–lowering effect. In 4 years of investigations, Dahl and other researchers discovered that the diet had *no* special ingredient. Instead, it was its very low salt content that made it work. When the same diet was used but with salt added, there was no beneficial effect on hypertension.

Dahl began to wonder. If low salt intake could lower blood pressure, might high salt intake be a cause of hypertension?

Over the next several decades, he worked with more than 32,000 rats. Thousands became hypertensive with chronic salt feeding. As the work continued, Dahl noticed that in unselected rats the response to salt ranged from no effect at all to gradually increasing blood pressures to rapid, severe elevations. About one-quarter of the animals showed no elevation, even after consuming a very high salt diet for most of their lives. The remaining three-quarters developed varying degrees of elevation, with 2 to 3 percent dying of hypertension after just a few months on salt.

This suggested genetic variances—hereditary influences.

Dahl then mated members at both extremes of the response range, producing two distinct strains of rats: a resist-

There may be people with so strong a genetic predisposition to hypertension that they need very little in the way of an inciting factor, such as salt intake, to develop it.

ant strain which could be fed a high-salt diet with no significant increase in average blood pressure—and a sensitive strain which showed significant rises in blood pressure with moderate salt intake and early death with high salt intake.

Dr. Dahl suggested, and many authorities now believe, that people react the same way.

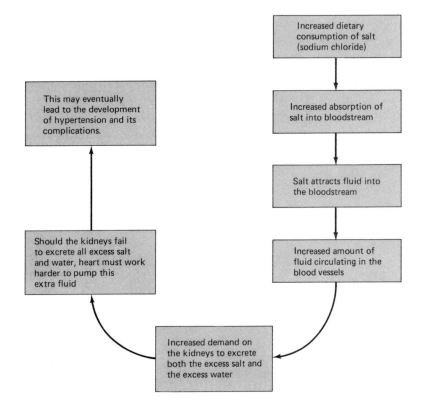

Salt: How it could affect blood pressure. (From Nutrition & Health 1 (3): 3, 1979.)

At one extreme, there may be people with so strong a genetic predisposition to hypertension that they need very little in the way of an inciting factor, such as salt intake, to develop it. At the other extreme, there may be people with no predisposition to hypertension, who do not develop elevated blood pressure even after eating high levels of salt all their lives. And there may be people with a slight predisposition, who may or may not develop hypertension depending upon how great their salt intake is.

Incidence of Hypertension

Many studies worldwide have found that among populations with minimal salt intake hypertension is rare; among those with high intake it is common.

Geographically diverse populations which exhibit virtually no hypertension and have low salt intake range from South Sea Islanders to Brazilian Indians to Alaskan Eskimos. In contrast, some populations with a lot of salt in their diets, such as the northern Japanese, have a very high incidence of hypertension.

Researchers recently studied residents of different villages of the Solomon Islands in the South Pacific. Most natives of the Solomons have not adopted the western custom

Correlation of average daily salt intake with proportion of hypertensive people in different geographic areas and among different races. (From Nutrition & Health 1 (3): 4, 1979; *adapted from J. D. Krudsen and L. K. Dahl,* Postgraduate Medical Journal 42: 148–152, 1966.)

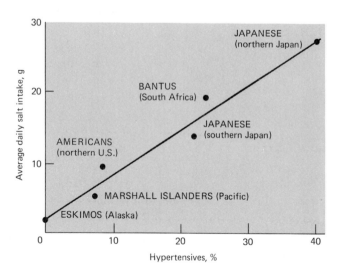

of adding salt to their food. In villages on the hill, the researchers found no high blood pressure and no rise of average pressure with advancing age, as occurs in the United States and all westernized countries.

In a village located on a lagoon, however, a significant incidence of high blood pressure was found, along with a rise in average pressure with advancing age. The lagoon villagers boiled their vegetables in seawater.

A Cutback for You?

Is there enough evidence to recommend that Americans should reduce their intake of salt?

As you have seen, many studies indicate that excessive salt intake is an important factor in hypertension, but none has absolutely proved the relationship. There may never be definitive proof, since that would require studying thousands of infants, half on lifelong salt restriction and half on the usual high-salt American diet, for as long a period as 30 to 40 years. Such a study would be virtually impossible to perform.

The evidence is strong enough, however, to convince many authorities that universal reduction of salt intake is justified.

To be sure, many people will never develop elevated blood pressure, even if they eat large amounts of salt all their lives. But others not now hypertensive will become so.

As yet, there is no way to predict who is and who is not susceptible; there are only some clues. Blacks, as a group, have a higher incidence; so do overweight people. A family history of hypertension increases the risk.

Since most Americans eat more salt than needed, it will do no harm and may do much good for all of us to reduce our intake of salt.

V.F., a successful Broadway producer, found that out the hard way. At 61 years of age, he developed a moderately elevated blood pressure of 155/95. His weight was normal, but his physician decided to have the EHE nutritionist evaluate his eating habits in relation to sodium intake.

His diet history revealed an excessive intake of salty

foods, particularly snacks. Because of the erratic nature of his profession, V.F. often skipped meals and would later grab a hot dog with potato chips or a sandwich (usually corned beef) and a pickle from a deli. He ate salted chips and nuts throughout the day for "energy." Despite his elevated blood pressure, he wanted to try dietary modifications first in order to avoid medication. The physician approved, and suitable low-sodium substitutions were made in his diet.

Today V.F.'s blood pressure is within normal range (less than 140/90), and he believes that even though it is difficult to adhere to the changes in his diet, they are worth the result he's achieved.

How Much Salt Are You Eating Now?

Americans love salt. Each of us on an average eats an astonishing quantity—$8\frac{1}{2}$ pounds a year, or 2 to $2\frac{1}{2}$ teaspoons a day.

In a review for the Food and Drug Administration, a committee of experts estimated American consumption as "not less than" 10 to 12 grams (equivalent to 2 to $2\frac{1}{2}$ teaspoons) of sodium chloride per person per day. Since salt is about 40 percent sodium, a salt intake of 10 to 12 grams means consuming at least 4 to 5 grams of sodium each day.

Many people are confused by the difference between sodium and salt. Health concern is with the *sodium* content of foods. Sodium occurs naturally in many foods and is also added via salt and other sodium-containing ingredients. Common among the latter are sodium nitrate (a curing agent and preservative), sodium benzoate (a preservative), monosodium glutamate (MSG, a flavor enhancer), sodium bicarbonate (baking soda, a leavening agent), and sodium phosphate (a wetting agent for quick-cooking cereals).

ABOUT SODIUM

Sodium in our diet comes not only from the salt we add to foods ourselves, but also from the salt and other sodium compounds (such as baking soda and monosodium glutamate) added to commercially prepared foods. In fact, salt is one of the leading food additives (after sugar)! The following list identifies some of the most important sodium compounds added to foods. While sodium is found in all of these products, it is the first five that are the major contributors of sodium to our diet.

- *Salt (sodium chloride)*. This is used in cooking or at the table, as well as in canning and processing.

- *Monosodium glutamate (MSG)*. MSG is sold under several brand names and is a seasoning used in home, restaurant, and hotel cooking, and in many packaged, canned, or frozen foods. It is often used generously in oriental cooking.

- *Baking powder*. Baking powder is used to leaven quick breads and cakes.

- *Baking soda (sodium bicarbonate)*. Baking soda is used to leaven breads and cakes; it is sometimes added to vegetables in cooking or used as an "alkalizer" for indigestion.

- *Brine (table salt and water)*. Brine is used in processed foods to inhibit growth of bacteria, as in corned beef, pastrami, pickles, and sauerkraut; in cleaning or blanching vegetables and fruits, and in freezing and canning certain foods.

- *Disodium phosphate*. This is present in some quick-cooking cereals and processed cheeses. It is used as an emulsifier in some cheeses and as a buffer to adjust acidity in chocolate products, beverages, sauces, and quick-cooking cereals.

- *Sodium alginate*. Sodium alginate is used in many chocolate milks and ice creams for smooth texture.

- *Sodium benzoate*. Sodium benzoate is used as a preservative in many condiments, such as relishes, sauces, and salad dressings.

- *Sodium hydroxide*. Sodium hydroxide is used in food processing to soften and loosen skins of ripe olives, hominy, and certain fruits and vegetables.

- *Sodium propionate*. Sodium propionate is used in pasteurized cheeses and in some breads and cakes to inhibit growth of mold.

- *Sodium sulfite*. Sodium sulfite is used to bleach certain fruits in which an artificial color is desired, such as maraschnio cherries and glazed or crystallized fruit; it is also used as a preservative in some dried fruits, such as prunes.

Sodium is not all bad. In fact, it's an essential nutrient without which we could not survive. It helps regulate blood and other body fluids and plays a major role in nerve-impulse transmission, heart action, and body metabolism of protein and carbohydrates.

A daily human sodium requirement is difficult to establish, because need can vary depending on such conditions as excessive sweating and diarrhea (which may require additional sodium). As a result, the National Research Council, rather than recommend a specific daily amount, has issued an estimate of an "adequate and safe" sodium intake for adults of 1000 to 3300 milligrams a day (1.1 to 3.3 grams), as compared with the 4 to 5 grams of sodium per day that Americans consume on an average.

In its report to the Food and Drug Administration, a committee of experts remarked: "It is the prevalent judgment of the scientific community that the consumption of sodium chloride in the aggregate should be lowered in the United States."

The committee's report added: "The average daily intake of sodium expressed as sodium chloride from all sources . . . exceeds estimates of the amount that may elicit hypertension in susceptible individuals."

The commissioner of the Food and Drug Administration, Arthur H. Hayes, Jr., M.D., recently met with representatives of 200 food industry associations to discuss lowering the salt content of processed foods. "We are looking into the need for new regulations," he said, "to require that the sodium content of food be declared on the label," adding that this was an important step to "help people help themselves to become healthier."

The Hidden and the Obvious

The salt that pours out of your salt shaker at dinner or during cooking accounts for only about one-third of all the salt in your diet. Some salt occurs naturally in food and in some drinking water, but up to one-half comes from processed foods.

According to information furnished to the Food and

The primary goal is to limit consumption of sodium. Like so many other elements of our diet, we eat too much of it. To begin to cut down, consider the following guidelines:

MAKING CHANGES

- To condition your taste to less sodium, gradually reduce the amount of salt you use at the table. Have your goal be to avoid adding any salt at the table. The conditioning takes approximately 2 weeks.

- To limit the amount of salt added when preparing foods, start cutting down by using just half the amount of salt called for in recipes.

- Be aware of "hidden" sodium in commercially prepared foods. Especially learn to avoid foods with MSG added to them.

- Season foods with herbs and spices instead of salt.

- Avoid or limit high-sodium foods. Use the list below as a guide.

Have:	Instead of:
Fresh or frozen vegetables (read labels for added salt; frozen vegetables vary in the amount of added salt)	Canned vegetables, sauerkraut, pickles, and food prepared in brine
Whole-grain or enriched breads	Breads, rolls, and crackers with salted tops
Fresh potatoes	Potato chips, canned potatoes
Unsalted nuts and pretzels	Salted nuts and pretzels
All fresh meats, poultry, fish, and shellfish	Cured, salted, canned, or smoked meats, poultry, and fish (e.g., corned beef, ham, bacon, luncheon meats, frankfurters, other sausages, sardines, anchovies, and marinated herring)
Unsalted or lightly salted homemade soup	Bouillon, canned or commercially prepared soups (especially Chinese soups)
Seasonings or spices and herbs	Soy sauce, catsup, garlic salt, onion salt, MSG, prepared mustard

From *Nutrition*, by Cheryl Corbin.

Drug Administration by one manufacturer, one serving of chicken or turkey noodle, tomato, chunky beef, vegetable beef, or cream of mushroom soup contains over 1000 milligrams of sodium.

Besides canned and dried soups, some other processed foods that contain large amounts of sodium are canned vegetables, cheese, tomato juice, dill pickles, olives, canned tuna and crab, sauerkraut, frozen dinners, and condiments such as soy sauce, catsup, and salad dressing. Items such as instant pudding, breakfast cereals, ice cream, cookies, cakes, and bread also contain significant amounts of sodium.

Laboratory analyses done for one consumer publication recently turned up some surprising information. You would expect salt in cocktail peanuts, but how about finding nearly twice as much sodium in a 1-ounce serving of corn flakes (260 milligrams) as in 1 ounce of peanuts (132 milligrams)? Or 234 milligrams in 2 slices of white bread versus 194 milligrams in a 1-ounce bag of potato chips? Or 404 milligrams in $\frac{1}{2}$ cup of chocolate-flavor instant pudding, 102 milligrams more than in a three-slice serving of bologna? Or 315 milligrams in just 1 tablespoon of a bottled Italian dressing, 1152 milligrams in a frozen fried chicken dinner, or 1510 milligrams in a Big Mac hamburger?

THE IMPORTANCE OF DIET

"When we consider the percentage of hypertensive patients who can be controlled with mild salt restriction (one-third of the mild cases, according to a recent Mayo Clinic study) and the percentage of obese hypertensive patients who can be controlled with weight loss alone (75% in our experience), we begin to realize what an important therapeutic weapon diet really is. . . .

"Perhaps the greatest challenge of the 1980's in the field of hypertension is not the development of new antihypertensive agents or new diagnostic procedures but of skills with which medical and paramedical personnel can motivate and guide patients in the nutritional management of obesity and hypertension."

Donald S. Silverberg, M.D.,
Hypertension Control Program,
General Federation of Labour,
Tel Aviv

SOME FOODS TO OMIT ON A SODIUM-RESTRICTED DIET

Food	Level of restriction		
	Mild	Moderate	Strict
Fruits	All forms are permitted (fresh, frozen, canned, and dried)	All forms are permitted (fresh, frozen, canned, and dried)	All forms are permitted (fresh, frozen, canned, and dried)
Vegetables, soups, and vegetable juices	Omit picked and dehydrated forms	Omit pickled and dehydrated forms Limit canned to 2 servings daily	Omit pickled and dehydrated forms Omit all canned and frozen if processed with salt
Meats, fish, poultry, and eggs	Omit cold cuts, sausages, and cured and pickled products	Omit cold cuts, sausages, and cured and pickled products Limit canned to 2 servings daily	Omit cold cuts, sausages, and cured and pickled products Omit all canned or frozen with salt
Bread and grain products	Omit salted crackers, pretzels, etc.	Omit salted crackers, pretzels, etc. Limit ready-to-eat and "quick cooking" cereals, commercial bread, or baked products to 3 servings daily	Omit salted crackers, pretzels, etc. Omit all products prepared with sodium
Milk and dairy products	Omit all cheeses and cheese spreads	Omit all cheeses and cheese spreads Limit fluid milk and milk products to 3 servings daily	Omit all cheeses and cheese spreads Omit all but low-sodium products
Seasonings	Omit bouillon, dehydrated soups, and soy sauce Limit salt to 1 tsp daily	Omit bouillon, dehydrated soups, and soy sauce Limit salt to $\frac{1}{4}$ tsp daily Omit catsup, mustard, commercial salad preparations, and seasoning salts	Omit bouillon, dehydrated soups, and soy sauce Omit all salt and salted butter or margarine Omit catsup, mustard, commercial salad preparations, and seasoning salts

SOURCE: *Nutrition & Health* 1(3):5, 1979.

How to Avoid Too Much Sodium

✱ *If you automatically use the salt shaker before you eat, stop yourself. Taste food before you add salt to it.*

✱ *Learn to enjoy the unsalted flavor of foods. They may taste different, but they are not tasteless. An acquired taste for salt can be changed.*

* *Ask the person who prepares food in your home to use as little salt and MSG in cooking as possible. Encourage, instead, the use of other seasonings in place of salt. Natural spices, herbs, and condiments such as pepper, parsley, chili, horseradish, and cloves contain only negligible amounts of salt and can be used liberally to make salt-free food tasty and satisfying.*

* *Replace salty snacks with unsalty ones, such as raw vegetables. Substitute peanuts in the shell for salted peanuts.*

* *Avoid canned soups or soup powders; they contain large amounts of salt (except for special brands of low-salt soup powders). In restaurants, avoid eating soup.*

* *Avoid eating canned, smoked, pickled, or cured meat and fish products as much as possible; they are usually high in salt. Preserved or pickled vegetables also almost always contain salt; frozen vegetables contain little or none.*

* *Ask the person in your home who shops for food to read labels carefully for additives containing sodium and to avoid products that list salt, sodium, or a sodium-containing additive near the top of the list of ingredients.*

REDUCING SALT INTAKE: DIETARY GUIDELINES

In general, a guide to ensure a diet balanced in the essential nutrients for an adult includes at least the following daily servings:

Dairy foods (milk, yogurt, unsalted cheeses)	2
Protein foods (meats, poultry, fish, eggs, and beans)	2
Fruits	4
Vegetables	3
Breads, cereals, pastas, and rice	4

The following meal suggestions apply to a moderate sodium restriction. When prepared at home remember to limit salt to $\frac{1}{4}$ teaspoon per day and select the appropriate foods as indicated in the preceding tables.

Breakfast: *Juice or grapefruit*
Eggs or unsalted cottage cheese
Toast
Unsalted butter or margarine
Cooked cereal (prepared without salt)
Milk (whole or skim)
Tea or coffee

A "brown bag" lunch: *Sliced chicken, lettuce, tomato, and alfalfa sprouts*
  on whole wheat bread
Raisins and nuts (unsalted)
Apple
Canned fruit juice, coffee, tea, or milk

A dieter's lunch: *Unsalted wafers or sandwich bread*
Hearty tossed salad (with everything in it except diced cheese
  and assorted canned vegetables, such as those served at
  salad bars) with vinegar and/or oil

Evening meal: *Broiled cod fish*
Broccoli with lemon sauce
Saffron rice (homemade without salt)
Dinner roll
Unsalted butter or margarine
Tossed salad
Fruit compote
Coffee, tea, or milk

Enhance your variety at home by making your own mayonnaise and salad dressing. When entertaining, dazzle your friends with some of these tempting items.

Dips: *Using yogurt as a base, stir in curry or black pepper, dill and*
  black pepper, or onion and garlic powder (not garlic salt).

"Dippers":   *Cherry tomatoes*
Cold, diced, cooked white potatoes
Fresh bean sprouts
Sliced green peppers, raw string beans, sliced carrots, sliced
  celery, etc.
Wafers and unsalted crackers, bite-size sandwich bread,
  pita bread

Gourmet favorites such as stuffed mushrooms, pastry puffs, escargot (snails), steamed seafood, meatballs, and aspics can still be served but should be prepared without salt. Dabble with such spices as coriander, cumin, fennel, ginger, and others you never thought of trying before. When serving dinner for a fancy occasion, convert your favorite recipes to salt-free versions. Vegetables are flavorful even when prepared without salt, and therefore should be incorporated more into menus.

When dining out, try to patronize restaurants that cook to order and prepare fresh vegetables, so that you will have more control over the amount of sodium in your food. Oriental restaurants use soy sauce, MSG, and pickled items; as a result their meals are inescapably high in sodium. Seafood and steak houses may offer some advantage if you can ensure that salt is not added during the preparation of your order. Salads and baked potatoes, which usually accompany such entrees, are quite safe if you forego the dressings and sauces.

Items from fast-food chains, and other deep-fried food selections, have a lot of added salt; here again a boiled or broiled version of the same food is a better choice.

Nutrition & Health 1(3): 4–5, 1979.

Executive Health Examiners Low-Sodium Diet

Most individuals eat more sodium than is necessary. Almost all foods contain some sodium. Following is a low-sodium diet which we prescribe for many clients. It is only mildly restrictive—limiting sodium intake to 2500 milligrams a day. Because of their natural sodium content, foods which are high in protein—such as meat, milk, and eggs—have been limited in this diet. The diet is nutritionally adequate, however, in that it provides enough protein, vitamins, minerals, and other nutrients required to maintain good health.

How to Use This Diet

The diet is divided into twelve food groups and includes one column for foods to be eaten on a daily basis and one column for foods to be avoided.

THE EHE LOW-SODIUM DIET

Food groups	Include daily	Foods to avoid
Milk	2 cups milk: condensed, whole, 2%, or skim.	Cultured buttermilk, instant cocoa or Dutch process cocoa, prepared beverage mixes, milk shakes, malted milk.
Meats, fish, poultry, eggs, and cheese	2 medium servings (9 oz total): fresh beef, lamb, pork, veal, fish, or poultry; low-sodium canned tuna or salmon, cottage cheese and low-sodium cheese. Limit of 2 oz regular cheese, 1 egg.	Any cured or processed meat or fish; kidney and brains; bacon; all sausage and lunch meat, such as bologna, chipped or dried beef; kosher meats; ham; frankfurters (hot dogs); canned tuna or salmon (unless salt-free); canned anchovies, caviar, herring, sardines; salted or smoked fish.
Vegetables	2 or more servings, fresh or frozen. (Low-sodium canned vegetables allowed.)	Regular canned vegetables and vegetable juices, frozen peas and lima beans, sauerkraut, olives.
Soups	Unsalted canned soup, unsalted broths, unsalted soups made with allowed milk and vegetables.	All others, including canned soups, bouillon cubes, broth, bouillon, frozen or dehydrated soup, regular soups.
Potatoes and substitutes	Any type without salt.	Potato chips, corn chips, pretzels, and salted popcorn; instant, packaged, frozen, and prepared potatoes.
Fruit	As desired: all fruit, frozen or canned.	Dried fruits containing sodium benzoate.
Bread	4 servings of regular bread. If more is desired, salt-free bread should be eaten.	Crackers, saltines, and pretzels.
Cereals	As desired: cooked cereals prepared without salt; puffed wheat, puffed rice, shredded wheat.	Quick-cooking and enriched cereals that contain a sodium compound; all other dry cereals.
Fats	6 servings: butter, margarine, cream, oils and shortenings, unsalted nuts, avocado, salt-free salad dressing.	Bacon, bacon fat, salted nuts, salted salad dressings.
Desserts and sweets	As desired: angel food cake, pure chocolate, cocoa, puddings and custard (if made with milk or eggs from day's allowance), gumdrops, hard candy, marshmallow meringues, mints, sugar. Limit 1 serving: regular bakery products (pie, cake, cookies, etc.) or ice cream.	Regular bakery products in excess of 1 serving daily; desserts made from milk in excess of allowance; any dessert with salted nuts.
Seasonings	Spices, herbs, lemon, pepper, vinegar. (See separate list below.)	Salt in all forms. Also, catsup, celery salt, chili sauce, garlic salt, horseradish, meat and vegetable extract, onion salt, prepared mustard, leavening agents, MSG, meat sauces (e.g., A-1), meat tenderizers, olives, pickles, relishes, soy sauce.
Miscellaneous	Coffee, tea, coffee substitutes, soft drinks except colas, gelatin, beer, wine, alcoholic beverages, unsalted nuts, unsalted popcorn. Limit of 12 oz cola beverage daily.	Cola beverages in excess of 12 oz daily, soda water, salted nuts.

Since foods must be prepared without added salt, they will be more flavorful if other seasonings are added. Here are some that you may want to try:

Allspice	Flavor extracts (vanilla, etc.)	Parsley
Anise	Garlic: whole, juice, or powder	Pepper: all types
Basil	Ginger	Poppy seed
Bay leaf	Leeks	Poultry seasoning
Beer	Lemon: juice or extract	Rosemary
Caraway	Mace	Saffron
Cardamom	Marjoram	Sage
Chili powder	Mint	Savory
Chives	Mustard, dry	Sesame
Cloves	Nutmeg	Sugar: brown or white
Coriander	Onion: whole, juice, or extract	Tarragon
Curry	Orange peel	Thyme
Dill	Oregano	Vinegar
Fennel	Paprika	Wine

Comments about your diet

Practice reading food labels. Avoid foods containing the following compounds:

Salt—in all forms
Sodium—in all forms
Baking powder
Baking soda (sodium bicarbonate)
Brine (salt and water)
Monosodium glutamate (MSG)

Caution: Ordinary canned vegetables almost always contain added sodium or salt without listing this information.

Daily meal plan

Breakfast:		Dinner:	
Fruit	$\frac{1}{2}$ cup	Soup	6 oz
Cereal	1 oz	Meat or substitute	6 oz
Egg (optional)	1	Potato	1
Bread	1 slice	Vegetable	$\frac{1}{2}$ cup
Fat	1 tsp	Fruit	$\frac{1}{2}$ cup
Milk	1 cup	Fat	1 tsp
Beverage	1 cup	Beverage	1 cup
Sugar	2 tbsp	Evening snack:	
Lunch:		Fruit	1
Meat or substitute	3 oz		
Potato	1		
Vegetable	$\frac{1}{2}$ cup		
Salad	1 medium		
Fruit	$\frac{1}{2}$ cup		
Bread	2		
Fat	1 tsp		
Beverage	1 cup		

LOW-SODIUM MENU

Meal	1	2	3	4	5	6	7
Breakfast	Orange and grapefruit slices Hot oatmeal with skim milk	Melon balls Pancakes with syrup	Papaya half Puffed wheat with skim milk	Pineapple slices Hot cream of wheat with skim milk	Peach Shredded wheat with skim milk	Fresh fruit and yogurt shake	Fruit compote with French toast
Lunch	Broiled hamburger on whole wheat roll with sliced peppers, onions, and cucumbers	Avocado stuffed with homemade lobster salad Zucchini bread	Turkey sandwich on pumpernickel bread Carrot-raisin salad	Mushroom omelet Marinated vegetable salad	Carrot bisque Peanut butter (no salt) and banana on bran bread	Roast beef sandwich on rye bread Potato salad	Cranberry juice Bagel with curried tuna fish (low-salt) salad
Dinner	Bluefish in white wine Cauliflower oregano Baked sweet potato Peach and blueberry pie	Coq au vin (chicken in burgundy wine with vegetables) Watercress salad Pineapple boats	Lamb and eggplant casserole Herbed brown rice Boston lettuce salad with honey poppy seed dressing Apricot fluff	Chicken breast marsala over whole wheat pasta Broccoli with lemon and garlic sauce Baked pears with candied ginger	Veal marengo with spaghetti squash Arrugula and endive salad Compote of poached fruit	Fresh mushroom soup Skewered swordfish Wild rice Herb baked tomato Cherries jubilee in meringue shells	Roast turkey with oat and mushroom stuffing Minted peas Baked apples with dates

Cholesterol

Cholesterol has come to be portrayed as a kind of coronary time bomb.

Virtually everywhere in the world that populations have been studied, those with high occurrence rates of atherosclerosis and coronary heart disease have been found to have high levels of serum (blood) cholesterol.

The reverse has proved equally true: among peoples with low serum cholesterol levels, the occurrence rates of atherosclerosis and coronary heart disease are low. In Japan, for example, where blood serum cholesterol levels average almost 100 milligrams per deciliter lower than in this country, the death rate from coronary heart disease is one-tenth our rate.

Many studies in the United States have shown that the risk of coronary heart disease rises sharply with increasing cholesterol levels. The Framingham study, for example, determined a frequency of disease seven times greater in persons with cholesterol values above 259 milligrams per deciliter than among those with values below 200 milligrams per deciliter.

If you could look into an atherosclerotic artery, the involvement of cholesterol would be obvious. You would find it as the chief fatty constituent of the fibrous fatty plaques that bedevil the vessel.

How Atherosclerosis Develops

Atherosclerosis used to be called *arteriosclerosis*, which translates literally as "artery hardening." *Atherosclerosis* is a more accurate descriptive term for the disease process, which starts with soft swelling (*athero-*) and then progresses to hardening (*-sclerosis*).

In a normal artery, a smooth lining of flattened cells (the *endothelium*) acts as a barrier to keep the blood and its contents flowing through the artery. Surrounding this lining, a thin sheath of muscle cells contracts or relaxes to control the artery diameter and help regulate the rate of blood flow.

When atherosclerosis begins, the earliest change visible to the eye is the development of fatty streaks—thin, slightly raised, yellowish lines—in the lining of the artery. These streaks are made up largely of cholesterol and cholesterol compounds (cholesterol esters).

As the disease progresses, the lining becomes thickened by soft deposits of fatty and cellular material called *atheroma* or *atheromatous plaques.* The cellular material consists of overgrown new muscle cells engorged with cholesterol. Damage to the artery lining causes the muscle cells to overgrow; one possible cause of damage is high blood pressure.

Studies in animals indicate that damage to the lining often is repaired spontaneously, but the damage persists or becomes worse when high blood cholesterol levels are present.

As disease progresses, the artery bore, or channel, is narrowed by the growing plaques and the scar tissue that may form around them. Blood flow is impaired. At some point, it may be cut off, and the area of heart muscle or other tissue normally nourished by the artery suffers injury or death.

Any artery can be affected by atherosclerosis, but those most often—and most seriously—affected are the larger vessels serving the heart, brain, legs, and kidneys.

The rate at which plaque develops varies considerably from one artery to another in the same person and from one individual to another.

The Long Buildup

Obvious manifestations of atherosclerosis rarely appear before age 40, because blood flow usually becomes seriously impeded only when there is more than a 75 percent narrowing of a vessel. The process begins in childhood, goes on slowly for years, and reaches an advanced stage in middle life or later, when manifestations appear, mainly as coronary attacks and strokes.

In the United States and other affluent western countries, one or more of the clinical manifestations affect one of every three men before age 60. In those countries, half of the annual death toll is traceable to disease of the heart and blood vessels, chiefly the result of atherosclerosis.

Women generally tend to lag 10 years behind men in developing manifestations of the disease, for reasons still not clearly defined. On undergoing menopause, they tend to lose their comparative immunity.

Cholesterol: Friend and Foe

Despite the bad reputation it has gained because of associations with atherosclerosis, cholesterol is a vital material.

It is contained in almost every cell in the body and may play a part in regulating the passage of nutrient materials into and out of the cell through the cell membrane.

It is found in high concentration in the brain and probably acts there in some important though not yet well-understood capacity.

Cholesterol is also a material from which many other important body materials are manufactured; for example, the corticosteroids, or hormones of the adrenal gland, such as cortisone, are derived from cholesterol. The sex hormones are derived from the sterol nucleus of cholesterol.

Cholesterol is also changed by the body to bile acids, which are excreted in the bile that flows into the intestine to help in the digestion of fats.

So a certain amount of cholesterol is essential, and the body produces its own as well as deriving some from food.

BLOOD CHOLESTEROL TESTS

Blood cholesterol tests are now an integral part of heart disease prevention programs, yet many physicians do not include them in your annual checkup. Your cholesterol level may be normal, but if you don't know, ask for a test. It's simple and requires only a blood sample that is sent to a laboratory for study.

The range between 125 and 220 milligrams per deciliter of blood serum is considered a safe cholesterol level by most cardiologists, but most middle-aged Americans (85 percent) have a cholesterol level well above 200 milligrams per deciliter. If this is true of you, you can begin to lower your cholesterol level today by eating more polyunsaturated and less saturated fats. Only a few months of careful eating will bring about an improvement.

CHOLESTEROL: ARE YOU AT RISK? EVALUATE YOURSELF.

	Blood cholesterol level	Body weight
Watch out	Above 260	Above 30%
	240–260	20%
Above-average coronary risk	220–240	10%
You're okay	175–220	0–9%

HDL and LDL: "Good" versus "Bad" Cholesterol

For many years, physicians were puzzled: Why did some people remain unaffected by atherosclerosis despite a seemingly dangerous level of serum cholesterol? Only recently has there been an explanation for this apparent paradox.

What is critical is not so much the total amount of cholesterol in the blood but rather how it is carried in the blood —the amounts of the various chemical "toters" of cholesterol, the substances which transport it in the blood.

Cholesterol is a fatty substance. Fatty substances do not mix with water, so the blood cannot carry them. In order to transport cholesterol and other fats from the liver to other organs and tissues, the body attaches them to proteins which are able to dissolve in blood.

Fats are known chemically as *lipids*, and the fat-protein combinations found in the blood are called *lipoproteins.* What has been known for some time is that there is more than one kind of lipoprotein—that, in fact, cholesterol is transported in two major types: high-density lipoproteins (HDLs) and low-density lipoproteins (LDLs).

As far back as 1951, one perceptive investigator, Donald P. Barr, M.D., of the Cornell University Medical College in New

York, considered that the two might not play the same role in atherosclerosis and that one, HDL, might be noninjurious, possibly even beneficial.

It was years before there was evidence for that. It came from the Framingham study.

As we noted earlier, for many years, starting in 1948, investigators have been closely following a group of more than 5000 men and women residents of this Massachusetts community, all healthy at the start. At the beginning of the study, the researchers noted facts about the residents' habits, lifestyles, blood pressures, and cholesterol levels, and they have been correlating such data with subsequent illnesses and deaths ever since then.

It was the Framingham study which established the significance of obesity, smoking, hypertension, and elevated cholesterol as risk factors for atherosclerosis.

In 1977, Framingham investigators discovered a striking new correlation: In virtually all of the 142 new cases of coronary heart disease which had developed in residents during the previous 8 years, HDL levels were low.

The average HDL level for American men is 45 milligrams per deciliter (about one-tenth of a quart) of blood plasma. For women, it is 55 milligrams.

Of the 79 men who developed coronary heart disease, 70 had levels below 45 milligrams, and of the 63 women, more than two-thirds had levels below 55 milligrams.

As William P. Castelli, M.D., laboratory director for the Framingham study, noted: "The most surprising finding of our study was the observation that the cholesterol contained in HDLs was inversely related to the incidence of cor-

---

What is critical is not so much the total amount of cholesterol but rather how it is carried in the blood—the amounts of the various chemical "toters."

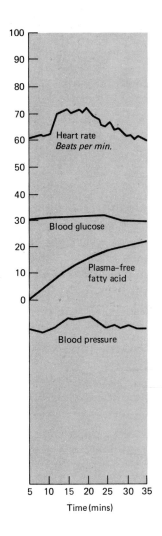

100
90
80
70
60 — Heart rate
       Beats per min.
50
40
30 — Blood glucose
20
10 — Plasma-free
       fatty acid
0

Blood pressure

5 10 15 20 25 30 35
       Time (mins)

THE EFFECT OF ONE CIGARETTE IN PATIENTS WITH CORONARY ARTERY DISEASE

One cigarette increases the heartbeat from about 77 beats per minute to 88 beats per minute, blood pressure increases slightly, and fats increase in concentration in the blood. These factors acting together cause the accumulation of fatty deposits in the arteries, leading to atherosclerosis and heart disease.

onary heart disease. As the HDL went up, the rate of coronary events went down."

More on HDL

The Framingham study and other investigations as well have found that newborn babies have about half of their total cholesterol in the form of HDL. But as they grow into adulthood and live a typically American life, the level of HDLs falls and that of LDLs increases.

Cholesterol: Friend and Foe   **129**

Women tend to maintain higher HDL levels longer than men, which may influence their lower rates of coronary heart disease. Eventually, however, increasing numbers of women, as well as many men, reach the point of having only about one-fourth of their cholesterol in HDL form.

In addition to the Framingham study, other recent studies—in Evans County, Georgia; Albany, New York; San Francisco; and Hawaii—have confirmed the importance of maintaining as high an HDL/LDL ratio as possible.

Moreover, C. J. Glueck, M.D., of the University of Cincinnati, has established that in families noted for longevity and freedom from heart and blood vessel disease, levels of HDL are very high—usually 75 milligrams or more per deciliter of blood plasma.

How does HDL protect?

Although more remains to be learned, LDL seems to be involved in transporting cholesterol to—and depositing it in—tissues, including blood vessel walls. On the other hand, HDL is apparently responsible for the reverse traffic, removing cholesterol from sites where it is in excess and carrying it back to the liver for disposal.

Thus it appears that HDL may act to thwart the atherosclerotic process by removing cholesterol from artery walls and helping to keep the arteries clear of deposits.

Raising Your HDL Level

Since HDL is good for you, how can you raise your HDL level?

* *Change your diet to one that emphasizes vegetables, cereals, and fish, with relatively little meat and no foods such as hot dogs and potato chips that are packed with saturated fats.*

* *Quit smoking and lose excess weight.*

* *Get more exercise.*

Studies of exercise often have found no great impact on total cholesterol and blood fat levels. However, at Stanford University Peter D. Wood, M.D., and his colleagues checked

The very active men had a lipoprotein profile much like that of young women largely free of coronary heart disease.

on forty-one very active men, aged 31 to 59. Many had not been particularly active earlier in life, but in the past year each had run at least 15 miles a week. They were compared with men of similar ages randomly selected from northern California communities.

The runners had an average total cholesterol level of 200 milligrams, compared to 210 milligrams for the other men—not much difference. But they had a much higher mean level of HDL—64 milligrams versus 43 milligrams for the others. The very active men had a lipoprotein profile much like that of young women largely free of coronary heart disease, rather than of sedentary middle-aged men.

A recent major study of 10,000 people at ten U.S. and Canadian medical centers, sponsored by the National Heart, Lung, and Blood Institute, examined the link between HDL and factors affecting coronary heart disease. The following observations were made:

* *Both smoking and obesity were associated with significantly lower HDL levels.*

* *HDL levels for smokers averaged 4 to 8 milligrams per deciliter lower than those for nonsmokers.*

* *Thin people had HDL levels 3 milligrams higher than those for people of average weight and height, and the average people, in turn, had HDL levels 3 to 4 milligrams higher than those who were obese.*

* *Moderate drinkers (about two mixed drinks a day) had higher HDL levels than nondrinkers. Among the drinkers, mean HDL levels were*

55 milligrams per deciliter, as compared with 42 milligrams for nondrinkers.

The Diet Influence

How strong is the evidence that a fat- and cholesterol-rich diet contributes to heart disease? Population studies have shown that in countries where the diet is rich in animal fats and cholesterol, the coronary death rate is much higher than where far fewer animal products rich in cholesterol and saturated fats are consumed.

The relationship is almost a direct proportion: the greater the cholesterol and saturated fat consumption, the higher the average serum cholesterol level and the higher the death rate from heart disease.

Studies of Japanese migrating to the United States have shown major jumps in serum cholesterol levels and heart disease after their arrival in America—evidently, researchers believe, because of the switch from an oriental to an American diet.

In animal experiments, monkeys fed a typically American diet have been found to develop coronary artery disease similar to that of human beings. Taking the monkeys off the American diet reversed the disease process.

Dietary studies in humans have shown that serum cholesterol can be predictably altered upward by an increase of saturated fats and cholesterol in the diet.

Other dietary studies have found that decreasing the proportion of calories obtained from saturated fats, increasing the proportion from polyunsaturated fats, and decreasing the amount of dietary cholesterol will lower the average serum cholesterol by discrete amounts.

Despite such studies, it has been difficult to demonstrate conclusively the relation of diet to blood fat levels and coronary heart disease in free-living Americans. Some investigations of Americans not placed on any special diets have failed to show any clear-cut direct relationship between diet and heart disease. Several reasons for this have been suspected. Most investigations have looked at only what the participants ate in a single day, yet there can be consider-

CHANGES IN CHOLESTEROL LEVELS AND RATE OF HEART DISEASE RELATIVE TO CHANGES IN DIET FOR JAPANESE MEN EMIGRATING TO THE UNITED STATES

	Japan	Hawaii	California
Diet:			
Calories, total	2164 ± 619	2275 ± 736	2262 ± 695
Animal protein, g	39.8 ± 22.8	70.5 ± 32.7	66.0 ± 24.4
Total fat, g	36.6 ± 20.4	85.1 ± 38.9	94.8 ± 36.4
Saturated fat, g	16.0 ± 13.3	59.1 ± 32.7	66.3 ± 30.5
Cholesterol, mg	464.1 ± 324.4	545.1 ± 316.4	533.2 ± 297.8
Blood cholesterol level:			
Milligrams per deciliter	181.1 ± 38.5	218.3 ± 38.2	228.2 ± 42.2
Level greater than 260 mg/dL per 1000 men	31.6	124.0	162.5
Incidence of heart attacks and/or death from coronary heart disease compared with incidence among Japanese men in Japan	—	2×	3×

SOURCE: Adapted from J. Stamler, "Population Studies," in R. I. Levy et al. (eds.), *Nutrition, Lipids and Coronary Heart Disease*, New York, Raven Press, 1979.

able variation from day to day in fat and cholesterol consumption. Procedures for measuring diet in people eating freely have not always been accurate.

New Evidence

A recently reported study which analyzed deaths among 1900 American men whose diets and cholesterol levels were first examined 20 years earlier provides new evidence of the importance of dietary factors.

Called the *Western Electric study*, the investigation was one of the largest and longest of its kind. Supported by the American Heart Association, the National Heart, Lung and Blood Institute, and other organizations and private donors, it was carried out by scientists of the Rush–Presbyterian–St. Luke's Medical Center, Chicago; the University of Michigan;

Harvard Medical School; and Northwestern University Medical School.

The 1900 men who took part in the study were employees of the Western Electric Company's Hawthorne works near Chicago. They ranged from 40 to 55 years of age at the start of the study.

For each man, a detailed dietary history was carefully taken—not just for a single day but for 28 days. More than 195 specific foods were reviewed to determine the number of times in the past 28 days each had been eaten and the usual size of the portions. Wax models of common foods and dishes of varying sizes were used as aids. Supplementary information about ways of preparing food was obtained by a questionnaire sent to each participant's wife. Restaurant meals were carefully checked.

Each man's diet was analyzed to determine usual caloric intake and consumption of animal and vegetable protein and fat, cholesterol, saturated and unsaturated fat, and vitamins. In each case, the blood cholesterol level was measured. A year later, the same procedures were repeated.

The status of the men was then checked on the twentieth anniversary of the first examination. It appeared that those who had had the lowest intake of cholesterol and saturated fats had a 33 percent lower death rate from coronary heart disease than the men with the highest intake.

As the investigators noted in their report of the study: "The results support the conclusion that lipid (fat and cholesterol) composition of the diet affects serum cholesterol concentration and risk of coronary death in middle-aged American men."

Richard B. Shekelle, M.D., senior author of the report, observed: "The message of these findings is that it is prudent to decrease the amount of saturated fats and cholesterol in your diet."

Proof and Prudence

Unquestionably, it would be nice to have incontrovertible proof of a cause-and-effect relationship between fat- and cholesterol-laden foods and atherosclerosis—to be able, for

> # The message of these findings is that it is prudent to decrease the amount of saturated fats and cholesterol in your diet.

example, to follow a molecule of cholesterol from its origin in an egg yolk to its final destination as part of an obstruction in a coronary artery. It would be highly satisfying, too, to have a very long term study—one in which, starting in childhood, thousands of individuals ate a low-fat, low-cholesterol diet—and to compare what happened to them in terms of atherosclerosis with what happened to others on a typical diet over half a century or longer. But we may not have the yolk-to-artery trail laid out for many years, and half a century is a long time to wait for results of any study from childhood on. Besides, such a study would be very complicated and expensive—perhaps too much so to make it possible.

Short of such proof, however, we do have mounting evidence that a prudent diet—one with reduced amounts of saturated fats and cholesterol—can be helpful.

In the opinion of Executive Health Examiners—as well as the American Heart Association, more than a dozen other organizations concerned with nutrition and health, and the U.S. Department of Agriculture and the Department of Health and Human Services—the magnitude and gravity of the problem of atherosclerosis do not permit indefinite temporizing while we await definitive proof.

Eating to Keep Cholesterol Levels Healthy

Dietary control of cholesterol levels in the blood is based on several principles.

The first is that foods differ markedly in their cholesterol content and cholesterol intake can be reduced by proper food selection. Among foods especially high in cholesterol

At only 27 years of age, how could W.V. already have a blood cholesterol level of 375 milligrams per deciliter? He was incredulous when the EHE physician told him this. Granted, he was not careful about the kinds of food he ate, but he did watch his weight. As a successful young stockbroker, he believed that being slim was all that mattered. However, the EHE physician reminded him, from his family history, that both grandfathers had died prematurely of heart attacks, and she advised him to see the nutritionist immediately.

W.V. had played football in college, and he had never stopped eating big, high-protein, high-fat meals like he had eaten when he was in training. When a low-fat, low-cholesterol regimen was planned for him, he found it wasn't too difficult to make changes gradually. One year later his cholesterol level is approaching normal (120 to 250 milligrams per deciliter), he is enjoying his new diet, and he can look forward to a long, healthy life.

are egg yolk (with 250 to 275 milligrams in a single yolk), butter (250 milligrams per 100-gram, or $3\frac{1}{2}$-ounce, portion), kidneys (375 milligrams per 100-gram portion), and sweetbreads (250 milligrams per 100-gram portion).

On the other hand, some foods have very little cholesterol content. Among them are fruits, vegetables, egg whites, cereals, vegetable oils, vegetable margarine, and peanut butter. Skim milk and milk powder are also low in cholesterol.

The second principle is based on the finding that the ratio between saturated and unsaturated fats in the diet is important in determining the blood cholesterol level. The lower the ratio, the lower the cholesterol level is likely to be.

When the association between high blood cholesterol levels and atherosclerosis was first noted, attempts were

The magnitude and gravity of the problem of atherosclerosis do not permit indefinite temporizing while we await definitive proof.

made to bring down cholesterol levels by reducing the dietary intake of cholesterol, but it turned out that reduced intake was not enough to bring the levels down to any marked extent.

Then it was found that the amount of *fat* in the diet matters. People placed on low-cholesterol diets but with fat intake still high continued to have elevated blood cholesterol levels. After considerable research it was found that fat in the diet seemed to facilitate the body's absorption of cholesterol in food.

However, it was determined that even low-cholesterol, low-fat diets do not invariably lead to blood cholesterol reduction. It took further research to establish that the *type* of fat consumed also counts.

There are, you may recall from an earlier chapter, three distinctive types of fats.

Saturated fats, which tend to increase blood cholesterol levels, are fats that harden at room temperature, such as gravy fat. Such fats are found primarily in foods of animal origin—meat and dairy products, particularly beef, lamb,

SOME RISK FACTORS RELATED TO DIET AND HEALTH THAT CAN RESULT IN HEART DISEASE

Risk factors*	Physiologic result	End result
Eating and drinking too much Not exercising enough	Overweight	
High total fat consumption High saturated fat consumption Low polyunsaturated/saturated fat ratio High cholesterol consumption	Elevated blood cholesterol	Higher risk of heart disease
High salt consumption Overweight	Elevated blood pressure	
Diabetes Smoking	Accelerates the atherosclerotic process	

* *Risk factors* are warning flags that suggest a greater-than-average probability of developing a related health problem. Most of the above risk factors are linked directly or indirectly to nutrition.
SOURCE: Select Committee on Nutrition and Human Needs, United States Senate.

pork, butter, cream, whole milk, and cheeses made from cream or whole milk. Saturated fats are also found in many solid and hydrogenated vegetable shortenings, such as coconut oil, cocoa butter, and palm oil, which are often used in commercially produced cookies, pie fillings, and non-dairy milk and cream substitutes.

Polyunsaturated fats, which tend to lower blood cholesterol levels, are fats that remain liquid at room temperature. Among them are such oils as corn, cottonseed, safflower seed, sesame seed, soybean, and sunflower seed.

Monounsaturated fats, a third type of fat, seem to have little, if any, effect on blood cholesterol levels. Olive oil is an example of a monounsaturated fat.

Applying the Principles of Cholesterol Control to Your Diet

You can probably apply the principles of cholesterol control to your present diet with moderate rather than drastic alterations.

Eggs Because egg yolks are so rich in cholesterol, a low-cholesterol, modified-fat diet to reduce elevated cholesterol calls for a maximum of three yolks a week, including those used in prepared food. There need be no limit on use of egg whites in cooking, since they are largely composed of protein.

Milk Products The fat in whole milk and whole milk products is saturated fat. To avoid that fat and still get the benefit of the protein, vitamins, and minerals, especially calcium, that make dairy products essential for your health, you can use skim milk and skim-milk products. Choose nonfat buttermilk, cottage cheese, and other cheeses low in fat (such as farmer and hoop) in place of high-fat cheeses (read the labels of cheese for fat—and sodium—content). In place of butter choose a margarine which indicates as its first ingredient a liquid polyunsaturated vegetable oil that is not hardened or hydrogenated.

Cream Sour cream is high in saturated fat; low-fat plain yogurt can be used instead in many recipes calling for sour cream.

Half-and-half is high in saturated fat and so, too, are many cream substitutes such as whipped topping and most nondairy creamers. They are made with saturated fats such as coconut or palm oil, so read labels carefully—don't assume that nondairy products can be substituted for dairy products if you are on a diet that excludes the latter.

Meat If you love steaks, chops, and roasts, you don't have to do without them entirely. But have them as entrees less often, eat smaller portions, and trim away visible fat. Dripping fat from roasts should be discarded rather than used for gravy. You can also eat less fried and more roasted, broiled, baked, and boiled meat.

Poultry and Fish As you cut down on steaks, chops, and roasts, you can eat more chicken and turkey; however, avoid their skin, which is where their fat is largely concentrated. You can also eat more fish.

Soup Eat soups if you like, but only those that do not contain a lot of fat. At home, much fat can be eliminated by refrigerating a soup after it is cooked and then skimming the fat off the top before reheating.

Fruits and Vegetables Eat more vegetables, salads, and fruits. Not only are they generally low in calories and fats and high in vitamins and minerals, but they also tend to moderate your appetite through their bulk.

Shortening When buying margarine, shortening, and prepared foods, check labels carefully. Beware of coconut and palm oils. Avoid items that list "hydrogenated" or "partially hardened" vegetable oils among the first ingredients on the label; they are saturated fats. Look for products that list polyunsaturated or monounsaturated liquid vegetable oil first.

Executive Health Examiners Low-Cholesterol, Modified-Fat Diet

Following are some guidelines which we prescribe for many executive clients to lower high blood cholesterol levels. They have proved practical and effective.

OFF THE SCALE AND UP ON THE TREADMILL

A substantial man—both in his company and physically—O.P. first turned up at Executive Health Examiners weighing 255 pounds! His blood cholesterol level, at 285 milligrams per deciliter, was too high as well.

He was all for doing something about his weight and cholesterol and, with little urging, undertook the EHE low-cholesterol, modified-fat diet.

He stuck with it and over the next 6 months lost 62 pounds. His blood cholesterol dropped down beautifully also—to 183 milligrams per deciliter.

One thing he did not do, though he had been urged to do it, was to significantly increase his physical activity, to get out and get some exercise—run, walk, or whatever, but exercise.

Even so, when O.P. was given another cardiac stress test, he had added 3 minutes to his endurance in 6 months. That was the result of having 62 fewer pounds to carry while walking briskly uphill on the treadmill.

No doubt he would have done even better with some physical conditioning, but still, for an overweight person, even without supplemental exercise, getting rid of excess weight can make a substantial difference by itself in physical endurance and tolerance for exertion.

Triglycerides

When most people think of blood fat damaging the arteries, they think of cholesterol, but other fat components, triglycerides, are also involved.

Triglycerides are compounds of glycerine and fatty acids. Most fat found in the body exists in the form of triglycerides, both when it is stored in tissues and when it is mustered to produce energy.

Just as cholesterol is always present in the bloodstream, so is triglyceride. The role of triglycerides in producing atherosclerosis is less well-defined than that of cholesterol, but there is evidence that high triglyceride levels are significant.

LOW-CHOLESTEROL, MODIFIED-FAT DIET: A LIPID-LOWERING REGIMEN

Foods to avoid	Foods to substitute
Butter, lard, most margarines	Safflower oil, corn oil, and other liquid vegetable oils (polyunsaturated), and margarine made from these
Coconut oil, palm oil	
Hydrogenated vegetable fats and oils	
Salt pork, suet, bacon, and meat drippings	
Gravies, unless made with allowed fat	
Sauces, unless made with allowed fat and skim milk	
Cream soups	Bouillon, clear broth, fat-free vegetable soup, cream soups made with skim milk, broth-based dehydrated soups
Salad dressings containing cheese and sour cream	Commercial mayonnaise
	Oil and vinegar
Whole milk, cream, sour cream	Skim milk, dried nonfat milk, yogurt made from skim milk
Most cheeses	Skim-milk cheese, cottage cheese
Fatty meats such as most cold cuts, corned beef, frankfurters, sausage, bacon, spareribs	Lean beef, lamb, veal, tongue, pork, and ham
Regular hamburger (ground beef)	Dried or chipped beef
Goose, duck, and poultry skin	Chicken, turkey (without skin)
Shrimp, fish roe (caviar)	Fish, except as excluded (if canned, drain oil)
Fried meats and fish, unless fried with allowed fat	Egg white; no more than 3 egg yolks per week, one of which may be replaced with 6 oz of shrimp or 3 oz of cheddar cheese
Meats, canned or frozen, in sauces or gravies	
Frozen packaged dinners	
Egg yolks (maximum 3 per week)	
Biscuits, muffins, sweet rolls, corn bread, pancakes, waffles, French toast	Whole wheat, rye, or white bread
	Saltines, graham crackers
Corn and potato chips, flavored crackers	Baked goods not containing excluded fat or egg yolk
Buttered, creamed, or fried vegetables prepared with excluded fat	Any vegetable, fresh, frozen, or cooked with allowed fat
Pork and beans	
Pies, cakes, cookies, other desserts containing excluded fats or egg yolks	Angel food cake, puddings, or frozen desserts made with skim milk, gelatin desserts
Ice cream, ice milk, whipped toppings	Water ices
Chocolate, coconut, cashews and macadamia nuts, most candies	Cocoa, nuts other than those excluded, hard candies, jam, jelly, peanut butter (old-fashioned type), honey, sugar
	Olives, pickles, salt, spices, herbs

In the Framingham study, triglycerides as well as cholesterol were found to contribute to the risk of atherosclerosis. The risk associated with one rose in proportion to the level of the other. Whether cholesterol was high or low, the risk rose with the level of triglycerides. The converse was equally true. People with high values for both seemed to be worse off than those with high levels of one or the other.

Like cholesterol levels, serum triglyceride levels are low in societies with a very low incidence of coronary heart disease, such as Japan.

The Normal and the Abnormal

Triglyceride levels below 150 milligrams per deciliter are in the normal range. Those between 150 and 300 milligrams per deciliter are in a gray zone, considered by many physicians to indicate mild abnormality. Levels above 300 milligrams per deciliter are considered to be definitely abnormal.

A word of caution: Hypertriglyceridemia (elevated triglyceride level) can be a real enough problem, but sometimes it can be a spurious one. When a blood sample is drawn to test for cholesterol, there is no need for your stomach to be empty, but for triglyceride testing, unless you have been fasting for 12 to 14 hours before blood is drawn, your triglyceride level will be falsely high. Because many patients are not aware of this, there may be unnecessary concern about spuriously elevated triglyceride levels.

Causes

In some cases, the elevation of triglycerides seems to be an inherited tendency. Much more often, however, abnormal levels are associated with excess weight. Excessive use of refined sugar and refined starches and excessive alcohol intake may also be involved.

Dietary Principles for Triglyceride Control

If your triglyceride level is abnormally elevated, it would be well to modify your diet according to three principles:

* *Achieve and/or maintain your ideal weight. Quite often, in obese people, weight reduction alone brings about a substantial decrease in elevated triglyceride levels.*

* *Reduce your intake of carbohydrates—particularly the simple carbohydrates found in sugars and products rich in sugar, syrup, and honey.*

* *Avoid excessive alcohol intake. Government studies indicate that the desirable maximum for daily alcohol intake is two drinks a day (2 ounces of liquor, or its equivalent in other alcoholic beverages).*

J.B., a 48-year-old dress buyer for an exclusive Manhattan department store, gained 15 pounds in the year between her physicals at Executive Health Examiners, making her a total of 75 pounds overweight. When the physician told her that her triglyceride level had risen to 415 milligrams per deciliter (the normal range is 30 to 150 milligrams), she decided it was time to lose weight for more than cosmetic reasons. Her aunt had developed adult-onset diabetes, and J.B. thought she might be a candidate, because elevated serum triglycerides can be a warning sign of diabetes. Moreover, her cholesterol level was high-normal for a woman her age, and the physician told her that a modified diet and weight loss would probably normalize both conditions.

The nutritionist worked with J.B. on a program of gradual dietary and behavior change over a period of 2 years, because at Executive Health Examiners we have learned that too many changes too fast are difficult for most people to

Often . . . weight reduction alone brings about a substantial decrease in elevated triglyceride levels.

CONTROLLED-CARBOHYDRATE, MODIFIED-FAT, MODERATELY RESTRICTED CHOLESTEROL DIET: A LIPID-LOWERING REGIMEN

Foods to avoid	Foods to substitute
Butter, lard, most margarines	Safflower oil, corn oil, and other liquid vegetable oils (polyunsaturated) and margarines made from these
Coconut oil, palm oil	
Hydrogenated vegetable fats and oils	
Salt pork, suet, bacon, and meat drippings	
Gravies and cream sauces containing animal fat	Vegetable oils, meat juices
Cream soups	Bouillon, clear broth, fat-free vegetable soup, cream soups made with skim milk, broth-based dehydrated soups
Salad dressings containing cheese or cheeses	Commercial mayonnaise
	Oil and vinegar
Whole milk, cream, sour cream, most cheeses	Skim milk, dried nonfat milk
	Skim-milk cheese, creamed cottage cheese, skim-milk yogurt (sugar-free)
Fatty meats, such as most cold cuts, bacon, sausage, corned beef, frankfurters, and spareribs	Lean, well-trimmed meats, such as beef, lamb, veal, pork or lean ham
Regular hamburger (ground beef)	Ground round or sirloin
Goose, duck, and poultry skin	Chicken, turkey (without skin)
Shrimp, fish roe (caviar)	Fish (if canned, drain oil)
Fried meats and fish, unless fried with allowed fat	Egg white, no more than 3 egg yolks per week, one of which may be replaced with 6 oz of shrimp, or 3 oz of cheddar cheese
Meats, canned or frozen, in sauces or gravies	
Frozen packaged dinners	
Egg yolks (maximum 3 per week)	
Biscuits, muffins, sweet rolls, corn bread, pancakes, waffles, French toast	Whole wheat, rye, or white bread
	Saltines, graham crackers
Corn and potato chips, flavored crackers	Baked goods not containing excluded fat or egg yolk, oats, bran
Buttered, creamed, or fried vegetables, unless prepared with allowed fat	Most vegetables, fresh, frozen, or cooked with allowed fat
Pork and beans	
Pies, cakes, cookies, other desserts containing excluded fat or egg yolks	Angel food cake, puddings, or frozen desserts made with skim milk, gelatin desserts (use in moderation)
Ice cream, ice milk, sherbert, whipped toppings	Water ices (preferably sugar-free)
Chocolate, coconut, candies, jams and jellies, syrups, honey, sugar	Any unsweetened fresh, frozen, or canned fruits or juices
	Most nuts, peanut butter (old-fashioned type)
Sweetened frozen or canned beverages	
Alcohol, except in small amounts	

make. When changes are gradual and based on established patterns, they are more acceptable and more often result in permanent alterations. This is what happened with J.B. Four years after achieving her weight-loss goal she has gained back only 5 pounds, and her serum triglyceride and cholesterol levels are normal.

Triglyceride-Control Diet

On page 144 are some guidelines prescribed for many executives, who have found it effective in lowering elevated triglyceride levels and maintaining control of cholesterol levels.

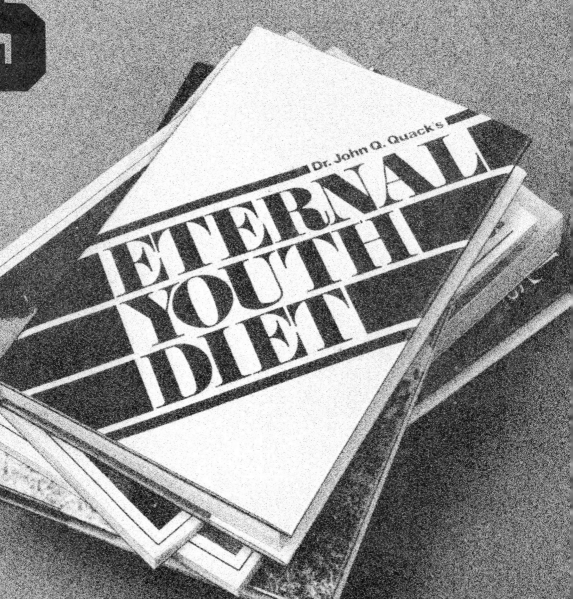

VITAMINS, MINERALS, AND FOOD FADS

If estimates are right, there are now 70 million Americans consuming an alphabet soup of vitamins and minerals every day. Many are taking doses hundreds or even thousands of times greater than required for good nutrition. The total expenditure for all these vitamins and minerals runs as high as $5 billion a year.

While some look upon these supplements as adding up to a kind of nutritional insurance policy, there are those who regard them as virtual panaceas for what ails them.

On these same grounds—nutritional insurance and nutritional therapy—consumption of other dietary supplements, such as alfalfa tablets, herbs and herbal brews, and "natural" and "organic" foods, has increased.

Claims and counterclaims about the benefits of taking supple-

Claims and counterclaims about the benefits of taking supplemental vitamins and minerals and of eating "health foods" have resulted in confusion and controversy.

*mental vitamins and minerals and of eating "health foods" have re-
sulted in confusion and controversy. Our aim in this chapter is to try
to help you separate fact from fancy on this topic.*

Vitamins

Casimir Funk, a Polish biochemist working in London in
1912 at the Lister Institute, originated the term *vitamine*,
which later became *vitamin*. Funk conceptualized the whole
idea that there exist certain vital nutrient accessory factors,
in the absence of which disease could result. No longer were
the causes of disease thought to be only foreign, noxious
agents; deficiencies of these necessary substances were also
considered as possible causes.

The idea of unknown vital substances in foods was not
without precedent. When Hippocrates prescribed liver for
night blindness in ancient Greece he was, although un-
knowingly, recommending vitamin A. When Quebec Indians
gave the scurvy-ridden men of Jacques Cartier a leafy brew,
they were dosing them with vitamin C. And when, in eigh-
teenth-century England, cod-liver oil was regarded as a
prized cure-all, it was because of its rich content of vitamins
A and D that made up for dietary deficiencies.

What Vitamins Are

Vitamins are organic molecules required in the diet in tiny
amounts to sustain the normal metabolic processes of life.
For the most part, they cannot be made in the human body.
There are, however, three exceptions. With adequate exposure to sunlight, you can produce vitamin D in your skin.
The B vitamin niacin can be synthesized from the amino
acid, or protein building block, tryptophan, and vitamin K is
made in significant amounts by bacteria normally present in
the intestines.

Vitamins function primarily as catalysts—action regula-
tors—in body chemical reactions. As such, they are essen-

Vitamins are required to sustain the normal metabolic processes of life.

tial for the release of energy, tissue building, and controlling the body's use of food. By themselves they supply no energy and build no tissue.

Each vitamin serves one or more special functions that no other nutrient can serve. Deficiencies of vitamins have specific results; in fact, part of the definition of a vitamin is that its lack produces a specific deficiency syndrome, or set of symptoms, and supplying it cures the deficiency.

One way of classifying vitamins is by their solubility in fat or water. The fat-soluble vitamins—A, D, E, and K—are stored in the body. Water-soluble vitamins—C, thiamine, niacin, and others—are not stored to any extent.

The amounts of vitamins required are very small and are measured in milligrams (one-thousandth of a gram) and micrograms (one-millionth of a gram; 28 grams equals 1 ounce) or in international units (IU). International units are used as a measure of the potency or ability of vitamins to promote growth, regulate metabolism or the processes of body maintenance, or cure a deficiency.

How Vitamins Work

Vitamins function as coenzymes. Once ingested, vitamins search out cells that need them and are taken into these cells. Within these cells, the vitamins combine with proteins called *apoenzymes*, which are already present there. The combination of vitamin and apoenzyme constitutes a *holoenzyme*—or *enzyme*, in short. It is the enzyme which serves the function of catalyzing or furthering specific metabolic reactions.

Why More Is Not Better

The critical function of a vitamin is to combine with the cell protein, the apoenzyme.

The quantity of any protein a cell can produce in a given time is limited. That limitation naturally applies to apoenzymes. Once the apoenzymes in body cells are saturated with a vitamin, no further activity can be achieved by adding more of it. The amount of a vitamin required to reach that saturation point is called the *recommended daily allowance* (RDA) of that vitamin.

The excess of a vitamin present in the body does not act as a coenzyme and therefore is not used to fulfill the positive functions of that vitamin. It may, however, become involved in other chemical processes that are harmful to the body. (This is discussed further later in this chapter.)

Recommended Daily Allowances (RDAs)

Early in World War II, the government became concerned about safeguarding public health by providing adequate supplies of essential nutrients. As a result, in 1941 the Food and Nutrition Board of the National Research Council of the National Academy of Sciences was established.

That same year the board, seeking a nutritional standard to use in measuring nutritional needs of groups of people, developed the first RDAs—designed, on the basis of available scientific knowledge, to meet the needs of almost every healthy person.

Periodic revisions—approximately every 4 to 6 years—have been made in the RDAs to incorporate new research findings. The RDAs are defined as . . . levels of intake of es-

A vitamin in excess may become involved in chemical processes that are harmful to the body.

THE ROLE OF VITAMINS

Vitamin	Functions	Deficiency symptoms
A	Aids in forming and maintaining the skin and the mucous membranes lining the intestinal tract and body cavities such as the nasal passages; also functions in visual processes to form visual purple and promote adaptation to dim light.	Night blindness, failure of bone growth, tooth decay, drying of eyes and mucous membranes and rough skin.
C (ascorbic acid)	Forms the cementing substances such as collagen that hold cells together, strengthens blood vessels, speeds wound healing, increases resistance to infection, and aids in utilization of iron.	Scurvy (hemorrhages, loose teeth, bleeding gums, poor or no wound healing, rough skin, muscle degeneration).
D	Helps in absorption of calcium from food in the digestive tract and building of calcium and phosphorous into bone.	In adults, osteomalacia (softening, deformation, and easy fracture of bones; muscular twitching and spasms); in children, rickets (growth retardation, bowing of legs, abdominal protrusion, malformation of teeth).
E	Helps to protect vitamin A and unsaturated fatty acids from destruction by oxygen.	Breakdown of red blood cells. (Although not found in humans, animals may show muscle disease, liver degeneration, failure of reproduction.)
K	Helps in blood clotting.	Hemorrhage.
Thiamine (B$_1$)	Aids in utilization of carbohydrates, promotes normal appetite, and contributes to functioning of nervous system.	Beriberi (heart swelling, leg cramps, mental confusion, muscle weakness).
Riboflavin (B$_2$)	Aids in the production of energy within cells and promotes healthy skin and eyes.	Eye sensitivity to light; cracks at corners of mouth; skin disturbances, particularly about nose and lips.
Niacin (B$_3$)	Contributes to the synthesis of fat, tissue respiration, and use of carbohydrates; fosters normal appetite; aids digestion; and promotes healthy skin, nerves, and digestive tract.	Pellagra (skin disorders, smooth tongue, mental confusion, irritability, diarrhea).
Pyridoxine (B$_6$)	Helps regulate use of protein, fat, and carbohydrates and assists in regeneration of red blood cells.	Skin disorders, cracks at corners of mouth, smooth tongue, nausea, dizziness, anemia, kidney stones; in infancy, convulsions.
Folic acid (folacin)	Aids in blood formation and contributes to the functioning of various enzyme and other biochemical body systems.	Anemia, smooth tongue, diarrhea.
B$_{12}$ (cobalamin)	Helps in blood formation and in maintenance of nerve tissues.	Pernicious anemia (appetite loss, intermittent constipation and diarrhea, abdominal pain, weight loss, tongue burning, irritability, depression).
Biotin	Helps regulate the use of carbohydrates and aids in the formation and use of fatty acids.	Symptoms not clearly established except under experimental situations, when appetite loss, nausea, fatigue, and depression have been noted.

RECOMMENDED DAILY ALLOWANCES FOR ADULTS

Nutrient	Adults		Principal food sources
	Male	Female	
Protein	56 g	46 g	Meat, poultry, fish, eggs, milk, hard cheese
Fat-soluble vitamins:			
Vitamin A	1000 μg RE*	800 μg RE*	Butter, yellow vegetables, liver, egg yolk, apricots, cantaloupe
Vitamin D	5 μg	5 μg	Butter, egg yolk, ultraviolet radiation (sunlight), fortified milk, liver, fish
Vitamin E (tocopherols)	5 mg†	5 mg†	Vegetable oils, wheat germ, cereals, legumes, egg yolk, green leafy vegetables
Water-soluble vitamins:			
Vitamin C (ascorbic acid)	60 mg	60 mg	Citrus fruits, tomatoes, strawberries, cantaloupe, green peppers, cabbage
Folacin	400 μg	400 μg	Green vegetables, milk, eggs, organ meats, nuts
Niacin	18 mg	13 mg	Whole grains, enriched bread, liver, meat, fish, poultry
Vitamin B_2 (riboflavin)	1.6 mg	1.2 mg	Milk, liver, green leafy vegetables, enriched bread and cereals
Vitamin B_1 (thiamine)	1.4 mg	1.0 mg	Enriched breads and cereals, wheat germ, liver, pork, nuts, grains, legumes
Vitamin B_6 (pyridoxine)	2.2 mg	2.0 mg	Pork, organ meats, fish, cereals, legumes, seeds
Vitamin B_{12}	3.0 μg	3.0 μg	Only foods from animal sources: liver, milk, eggs, meat
Minerals:			
Calcium	800 mg	800 mg	Milk, cheese, soybeans, greens
Phosphorus	800 mg	800 mg	Liver, meat, poultry, milk, wheat germ, legumes, nuts
Iodine	150 μg	150 μg	Iodized salt, ocean fish
Iron	10 mg	18 mg	Liver, meat, eggs, wheat germ, enriched cereals and breads, green vegetables
Magnesium	350 mg	300 mg	Nuts, legumes, soybeans, green leafy vegetables
Zinc	15 mg	15 mg	Seafood, nuts, meat, eggs, green leafy vegetables

* Retinol equivalents.
† Approximately equal to total vitamin E activity.
SOURCE: *Recommended Dietary Allowances, Revised 1980,* Food and Nutrition Board, National Academy of Sciences, National Research Council, Washington.

sential nutrients considered . . . on the basis of available scientific knowledge . . . to be adequate to meet the known nutritional needs of practically all healthy persons. . . . They are recommendations for maintaining health but do not cover specific needs due to illness. They are recommendations for amounts of nutrients which should be consumed—that is, actually eaten—and make no allowances for any amounts that may be lost during processing or food preparation.

How Well Do Foods Meet the RDAs?

Eat one medium-sized baked sweet potato, or half a cup of peas and carrots, or the same quantity of spinach to satisfy the RDA for vitamin A.

For vitamin C, eating a medium-sized stalk of broccoli (about 6 ounces), or half of a 5-inch cantaloupe, or half a cup of frozen orange juice will satsify the RDA.

Eating 3 ounces of either pork, calf, or beef liver will supply all the riboflavin that is needed. Or drinking 2 cups a day of milk (low-fat, whole, or skim) will meet about half the RDA.

Three ounces of pork liver supplies the RDA of niacin. Three ounces of waterpacked tuna or the same amount of turkey or chicken (roast breast) will contribute about half of the RDA.

These few examples indicate why it is often said that anyone who eats a well-balanced diet usually needs no added vitamins. Such a diet includes daily at least four servings of grain and cereal products, four or more of a variety of fruits and vegetables, two servings of dairy products, and two of meat, fish, or poultry.

Who Needs Vitamin Supplements

Unfortunately, not all of us eat a well-balanced diet. Some of us eat erratically, others eat very low calorie diets, and then there are picky eaters whose diets are quite limited. For such people, multivitamin pills may be indicated.

There are people with special problems who may need vitamin supplementation—those, for example, who have a disorder of absorption; others who require extra amounts of pyridoxine because of a genetically induced imbalance.

There are some people who believe in "nutritional insurance" to the extent of taking a capsule a day containing the RDAs of major vitamins. Many physicians have no quarrel with that. They consider, as one puts it, that it is "totally unnecessary, but if it makes someone feel better, he or she is out only a couple of cents a day."

Megavitamin doses, however, are another matter.

What Are Megavitamin Doses Supposed to Do, and Do They Do It?

Many claims have been made, and continue to be made, for the values of vitamins in large doses. Megadoses—particularly of vitamins C and E—are said by some to be effective for ills that the ordinary diet cannot handle. Consistently, however, the claimed benefits have failed to stand up under close scientific scrutiny.

Vitamin C The idea that increased intake of vitamin C may be useful for the common cold has been around since the 1930s, although it gained widespread popularity only in 1970 with the publication of Dr. Linus Pauling's best-seller, *Vitamin C and the Common Cold.*

It has been suggested that large doses of vitamin C can prevent colds or can cure them once they have begun, but many carefully controlled experimental studies have failed to support these claims.

Are there any benefits at all to taking large doses of vitamin C? One of the major independent investigators, Terence W. Anderson, M.D., of the University of Toronto, has suggested that increased regular intake of vitamin C or a larger therapeutic dose (not of the order of grams but about 100 to 150 milligrams a day) at the time of illness "may have a small beneficial effect and this effect appears to be on severity rather than on frequency or total duration of colds."

Many claims have been made, and continue to be made, for the values of vitamins in large doses.

It has been suggested that large doses of vitamin C can prevent colds or can cure them once they have begun.

ESTIMATED SAFE/ADEQUATE DAILY INTAKES OF ADDITIONAL SELECTED VITAMINS AND MINERALS

Nutrient	Adults	Principal food sources
Vitamins:		
Vitamin K	70–140 μg	Spinach and greens, broccoli, cauliflower, vegetable oils
Biotin	100–200 μg	Organ meats, mushrooms, peanuts
Pantothenic acid	4.0–7.0 mg	Organ meats, yeast, eggs, salmon, broccoli, mushrooms
Trace elements:		
Copper	2.0–3.0 mg	Shellfish, organ meats, nuts, legumes, raisins
Manganese	2.5–5.0 mg	Nuts, legumes, whole grains, tea
Fluoride	1.5–4.0 mg	Drinking water
Chromium	0.05–0.2 mg	Whole grains, brewer's yeast, animal products
Selenium	0.05–0.2 mg	Grains and onions
Molybdenum	0.15–0.5 mg	Cereals, legumes, beef kidney
Electrolytes:		
Sodium	1100–3300 mg	Table salt, processed foods
Potassium	1875–5625 mg	Meats, fruits, juices, vegetables, legumes, cereals
Chloride	1700–5100 mg	Table salt, processed foods

SOURCE: *Recommended Dietary Allowances, Revised 1980,* Food and Nutrition Board, National Academy of Sciences, National Research Council, Washington.

Is further study warranted? Some investigators think not, arguing that although vitamin C may have a slight effect on the common cold, it is too small to be of any practical value and the subject is not worth pursuing.

Dr. Anderson is one of those who are open-minded on the subject, and he favors continued study. "It is possible," he notes, "that if we fully understood the mechanism involved in producing even a slight effect, we might be able to develop it further and produce effects that were quantitatively more worthwhile."

More recent claims that vitamin C can help cancer patients have thus far not been confirmed. In a clinical trial at the Mayo Clinic in Rochester, Minnesota, high doses of vitamin C gave no indications of prolonging or improving the lives of terminally ill cancer patients.

Vitamin E Claims have been made that large doses of this vitamin can promote physical endurance, enhance sexual potency, treat menopausal disturbances, prevent heart attacks and a variety of heart and blood vessel diseases, slow down aging, and act against such disorders as muscular dystrophies, cystic fibrosis, and diabetes.

But these claims have not been substantiated.

Vitamin E supplements are valuable for a rare type of anemia in babies and in individuals with intestinal disorders in which absorption is impaired. In Baltimore, a group of investigators led by Robert S. London, M.D., reports that vitamin E may play a role in the treatment of fibro-cystic breast disease, but cautions that it must not be taken for this condition except under a physician's supervision.

What Harm Can Megadoses Do?

For some vitamins, notably A and D, the harm of overdosing has long been appreciated.

In excess, vitamin A can be poisonous. The symptoms of poisoning can be variable—restlessness, appetite loss, weight loss, hair loss, muscle pains, swelling over long bones, headache, and generalized weakness, with death as a possible result.

For some vitamins, notably A and D, the harm of overdosing has long been appreciated.

Too much vitamin D can lead at first to such symptoms as appetite loss, nausea, and vomiting, followed by weakness, nervousness, itching, extreme thirst, and frequent uri-

VITAMIN TOXICITIES: THE OLDEST KNOWN, A, AND MOST COMMON, D

Ever since 1857, when Arctic explorers ate large amounts of polar bear liver, which is rich in vitamin A, the curious syndrome of acute toxicity—headache, dizziness, and diarrhea—caused by ingesting excessive amounts of vitamin A has been known. It is now recognized that the symptoms are caused mainly by increased fluid pressure within the brain and spinal column.

Although sometimes prescribed for certain skin conditions in carefully regulated doses, *chronic* excessive intake of vitamin A results in a cirrhosis-like liver condition. It can also lead to abnormal bone changes.

Vitamin D, which recent research has established is actually a hormone rather than a vitamin, has earned the reputation of being responsible for more serious toxicity than any other vitamin.

Once there was a long period of enthusiasm for treating rheumatoid arthritis with large vitamin D doses, leading in many cases to calcinosis (abnormal deposits of calcium in tissues).

Continued intake of 50,000 units of vitamin D a day is enough to cause poisoning, manifested in the early stages by weakness, fatigue, lassitude, headache, nausea, vomiting, and diarrhea. Later, kidney function becomes impaired, leading to excessive thirst, frequent urination and the loss of protein in the urine. Still later, there may be kidney stones, and eventually all soft tissues of the body are invaded by calcium salts, while the bones lose their normal density and become fragile.

> Vitamin D, which recent research has established is actually a hormone rather than a vitamin, has earned the reputation of being responsible for more serious toxicity than any other vitamin.

nation. With continued intake of excessive amounts of the vitamin, kidney function can be impaired.

What of such vitamins as C and E? Although it has been alleged that megadoses of them are harmless, there is a growing body of evidence that this is not true.

You will recall that excess vitamins can become involved in chemical reactions besides those associated with their primary functions. In megadoses, the quantities are so great that the enzyme systems in which they are incorporated become saturated. The megadose excess is then free to become involved in other chemical reactions.

Thus excess vitamin C, for example, may raise the level of uric acid in the urine and trigger gout in predisposed people. It has been reported, as well, that in some people excess vitamin C can lead to an increased susceptibility to kidney stones.

Rebound scurvy may be another undesirable effect. It develops when the body, exposed to the chemical effects of excess vitamin C, speeds up its machinery for destroying the vitamin excess. If this happens in a pregnant woman, the fetus may acquire the same speeded-up machinery and may be born with a vitamin C–destructive capacity much greater than normal. The newborn may then develop scurvy, which could result in dangerous, even life-threatening, bleeding.

Similar but less dangerous rebound scurvy has been reported in adults who stop megadoses of vitamin C abruptly rather than cut back slowly at a rate of about 10 percent a day. They may develop bleeding of the gums and under the skin, loosening of the teeth, and roughening of the skin.

For some people—about 13 percent of American blacks

and as many as 20 percent of Sephardic Jews, Orientals, and some other ethnic groups—megadoses of vitamin C may present another danger. These people have a genetic abnormality—a deficiency in the enzyme glucose-6-phosphate dehydrogenase (G6PD). Ordinarily the deficiency produces no symptoms whatever and causes no problems, except under circumstances involving the use of certain drugs or in the presence of severe infection. Then it may cause the destruction of many red blood cells and anemia.

Some years ago there was a mystery about an anemia that developed in some members of the armed forces who were under treatment with drugs to overcome or prevent malaria. The anemia was being caused by the drugs, which helped many others but were harmful to these men because they had a G6PD deficiency. When this was discovered, the antimalarial drug dosage was adjusted so it produced only mild red-cell destruction in the susceptible individuals.

Subsequently, it became known that in the presence of G6PD deficiency, anemia may be produced by other drugs such as aspirin, sulfa compounds, phenacetin (which is found in some headache remedies), and nitrofurantoin (an antibacterial agent used in treating some urinary tract infections). Still more recently, there have been reports that megadoses of vitamin C may lead to severe anemia in susceptible individuals with G6PD deficiency, and at least one death has been reported.

These are not the only undesirable effects that megadoses of vitamin C may have.

At the Bronx Veterans Administration Medical Center studies indicate that megadoses of vitamin C can destroy half or more of the vitamin B_{12} in a typical VA Hospital diet.

Diabetics checking their urine may get false negative results from one test (Testape) and false positive results from another (Clinitest) because of the effects of large doses of vitamin C, thus increasing the risk of either diabetic ketoacidosis or insulin shock.

Recent reports also indicate that megadoses of vitamin C can cause false negative results of tests for blood in the stool —a means of detecting cancer of the colon.

What are the undesirable effects of vitamin E megadoses? Those reported so far include headaches, nausea, fatigue, and dizziness. Blurring of vision also has been reported, and there is some suspicion that this may occur because large doses of vitamin E antagonize vitamin A.

Megadoses of vitamin E also have been reported to cause inflammation of the mouth, chapping of the lips, muscle weakness, low blood sugar, gastrointestinal disturbances, and increased bleeding.

Because she didn't have "time to eat," M.L., a 30-year-old

"VITAMIN B₁₅"— WHATEVER IT IS, IT WON'T HELP

A so-called vitamin sold in health food stores may be giving users cancer rather than prolonging their lives, according to a report in the *Journal of the American Medical Association*.

One of the components of "vitamin B_{15}," also known as calcium pangamate or pangamic acid, has been found by Neville Colman, M.D., of the Bronx Veterans Administration Medical Center, New York, to be mutagenic (capable of causing mutations) in a widely used laboratory test. A chemical that is mutagenic in this test has a 90 percent probability of being able to cause cancer, Dr. Colman notes.

Vitamin B_{15} is promoted as a dietary supplement as well as a drug. According to the Food and Drug Administration, it has been alleged to help heart disease, aging, diabetes, gangrene, hypertension, glaucoma, alcoholism, hepatitis, jaundice, allergies, dermatitis, neuralgia, and neuritis.

After mixing 6-demethyl griseofulvin (DMG), a compound found in the largest selling formulation of vitamin B_{15}, with a chemical to simulate exposure to saliva and incubating the mixture under conditions similar to those in the human stomach, Colman and his colleagues concluded that the compound is capable of reacting to form a potential carcinogen under conditions simulating those found in the human digestive tract.

The discovery of pangamic acid was announced in 1943 by Ernst Krebs, Sr., and Ernst Krebs, Jr. (who gave the world laetrile). They applied for a patent and said they had isolated the material from apricot kernels. After the patent was granted in 1949, the material was heavily promoted as a cure-all under the trade name vitamin B_{15}.

Journal of the American Medical Association 243:2473, 1980.

junior partner in a law firm, took vitamin supplements—lots of them. She believed they would compensate for her poor diet and help relieve the enormous pressure she was under all the time.

When she visited the EHE nutritionist, she brought with her a sheet from a legal pad divided into two columns, completely filled with the names of the miscellaneous "nutrients" she took at intervals throughout the day. However, instead of feeling better, each day she felt worse.

Was there something else she should be taking?

She had heard that megadoses of vitamin C might cause kidney stones in susceptible people, and having had stones once ("It was very uncomfortable") she did not want to have them again.

The nutritionist helped M.L. to realize that these supplements were no substitute for an adequate diet and that they could not combat the psychological stress she was undergoing on the job. He pointed out that the liquid potassium supplement she was taking was potentially dangerous and should not be consumed without a physician's supervision, even though she was able to purchase it without a prescription.

M.L. was weaned from most of her self-prescribed supplements, and she gradually began to eat more balanced meals and snacks and to feel more energetic. This, in turn, improved her ability to withstand the stress of her job and started her on the way to a healthier lifestyle.

Not everyone takes megadoses of vitamins to compensate for improper nutrition. Some people take liquid protein.

At age 42, T.C., an insurance broker, had a problem: he did not know *how* to eat. He had always been obese until last year, when he entered a community weight-loss program that combined fasting with taking liquid protein.

The program, not considered entirely safe by most physicians, is *not* endorsed by Executive Health Examiners. Of course, it worked in a way for T.C. After all, a person who does not eat for months at a time is bound to lose weight. T.C. did lose 95 pounds because of the severely restricted intake of this diet, but he had not learned what he *could* eat so that he would not gain all of it back. He had already regained 15 pounds and was extremely discouraged when he first entered the EHE nutrition program. Before he came to Executive Health Examiners, he had even considered beginning one of the country's most popular fad diets of high protein and low carbohydrate intake, which allows a person to eat all the meat and fatty foods he or she desires but severely limits the intake of fruits and starches.

The nutritionist discouraged T.C. from following this diet, especially after examining his laboratory report which showed slightly elevated cholesterol and uric acid levels that could have been further aggravated by the high fat and protein components of the diet.

One of the nutritionist's first steps was to assure T.C. that the common belief that complex carbohydrates are more fattening than similar portions of meat is incorrect and to convince him that most nutritionists recommend increased consumption of these complex carbohydrates for improved health. Because T.C.'s favorite foods included complex carbohydrates such as pasta and whole-grain breads, it would have been unwise for him to have restricted them severely.

Subsequently, a system of daily food record keeping, dietary guidelines based on favorite foods, and monthly visits to Executive Health Examiners for reinforcement was established. It has proved very successful, and T.C. has finally learned *how* to eat.

Minerals

Among the 40-odd nutrients known to be essential to man —including carbohydrates, fats, amino acids, and vitamins —are more than a dozen minerals. Two essential minerals alone, calcium and phosphorus, represent 3 percent of total body weight.

Minerals are elements found in water and food that are required as structural components and as participants in many of the body's vital processes. Those minerals which are needed by the body are often classified, in terms of the relative quantities required, as either *macro*nutrients (required in large amounts) or *micro*nutrients (required in small amounts). Micronutrients, in fact, are often called *trace elements* because they are needed in such small amounts.

Better from a Pill? An Example of Why Not

Zinc supplementation recently has become popular. Certainly, it is an important mineral. Recent research indicates that it is a constituent of more than 80 enzymes involved in many metabolic processes, such as growth, reproduction, and disease resistance. Along with other trace elements, it is believed by some to have a protective effect against heart disease.

The adult RDA of zinc, as set by the Food and Nutrition Board of the National Academy of Sciences, is 15 milligrams a day. The board has advised that supplements should not exceed that amount by more than 15 milligrams a day; however, zinc supplements found in health food stores and elsewhere include dosages of 10, 22, 30, 50, and 100 milligrams!

Is there a potential danger from excessive amounts of zinc?

At a recent New York Academy of Sciences symposium, Dr. Walter Mertz of the U.S. Department of Agriculture Nutrition Institute, noted: "At a certain level, not overly high, zinc can interact with other essential trace elements, notably copper. You can produce a relative copper deficiency."

At the same symposium, Leslie Klevay, M.D., a medical researcher at a Department of Agriculture human nutrition laboratory, told of experiments with rats which showed that high blood cholesterol levels could be produced by increasing the amount of dietary zinc relative to copper. Subsequently, when the zinc/copper ratio was decreased, cholesterol levels fell, as did the death rate among the animals.

Zinc supplementation recently has become popular. Is there a potential danger from excessive amounts of zinc?

By producing a relative deficiency of copper, could excessive intake of zinc be a threat to human beings?

Dr. Klevay reported:

> There are many similarities between people with atherosclerosis and ischemic heart disease and animals deficient in copper. A member of either group is likely to die suddenly, to be hypercholesterolemic [have high blood cholesterol levels] and hyperuricemic [have high urinary uric acid levels], to have arteries with abnormal connective tissue and to have fibrotic, hypertrophied [abnormally large] hearts low in copper, with abnormal electrocardiograms.

The zinc-copper interaction is just one example of how it is possible, through indiscriminate supplementation, to distort the physiological ratio between various minerals and actually cause a mineral deficiency.

Another reason for care in supplementation, where it may be indicated, is that an excess of a particular mineral can sometimes have a direct, hazardous effect.

Below is a guide to the mineral nutrients.

Calcium and Phosphorus

These two minerals often work together. Both are involved in the formation of bones and teeth, and both are needed for normal functioning of the nervous system. Phosphorus goes into the making of the chemical adenosine triphosphate (ATP), which is sometimes referred to as a kind of "body spark plug" because, in effect, it sparks the release of energy from glucose for such activities as muscle movement.

Calcium is needed for normal blood clotting, and phosphorus is required for the metabolism of some carbohydrates.

A persistent deficiency of calcium can lead to bone deterioration, including osteoporosis, a thinning of bone structure that affects some men and as many as one-fourth of postmenopausal women.

Milk and dairy products are especially good sources of calcium, not only because of their high content of this mineral but also because milk sugar, lactose, enhances calcium absorption from the intestine. The RDA for calcium for

SOME CALCIUM-RICH FOODS

Food	Serving	Calcium content, mg
Sardines with bones	3 oz	372
Skim milk	1 cup	296
Whole milk	1 cup	288
Yogurt	1 cup	272
Cheddar cheese	1 oz	213
Oysters	$\frac{3}{4}$ cup	170
Canned salmon with bones	3 oz	167
Collard greens	$\frac{1}{2}$ cup	145
Creamed cottage cheese	$\frac{1}{2}$ cup	116
Spinach	$\frac{1}{2}$ cup	106
Ice cream	$\frac{1}{2}$ cup	97
Mustard greens, cooked	$\frac{1}{2}$ cup	97
Corn muffins	1	96
Kale, cooked	$\frac{1}{2}$ cup	74
Broccoli stalks, cooked	$\frac{1}{2}$ cup	68
Oranges	1 medium	54

adults is 800 milligrams a day, and 2 cups of milk (either skim or whole) can supply about two-thirds of this requirement. Sardines with bones are another rich source of calcium.

Vitamin D—produced in the skin by sunlight and contained in fortified margarine and milk products—is needed for calcium absorption, too.

THE CALCIUM-TO-PHOSPHORUS RATIO

The ideal ratio of dietary calcium to phosphorus is considered to be 1.5 to 1 in infants up to 6 months of age, 1.35 to 1 in infants between 6 months and 1 year in age, and 1 to 1 in older children and adults. Phosphorus intake is much higher than that of calcium for most Americans because phosphorus is more abundant than calcium in most foods.

Calcium and phosphorus content of 100-gram portions of selected food items and their calcium/phosphorus ratio

Food item	Calcium, mg	Phosphorus, mg	Ca/P ratio
Beef liver	8	352	1:44
Gatorade	0.2	7	1:35
Pork loin	12	234	1:20
Chicken breast	11	214	1:19
Bologna	32	581	1:18
Fish (flounder, sole)	12	195	1:16
Flour, whole wheat	41	372	1:9.1
Potatoes	7	53	1:7.6
Peanuts	69	401	1:5.8
Coca-Cola	3	16	1:5.3
Peas, green	26	116	1:4.5
Rice, white	24	94	1:3.9
Eggs	54	205	1:3.8
Beans, white	144	425	1:3
Almonds	234	504	1:2.2
Cottage cheese	94	152	1:1.6
Processed cheese	697	771	1:1.1
Milk, cow's	118	93	1:0.8
Beans, green	56	44	1:0.8
Cheddar cheese	750	478	1:0.6
Spinach, fresh	93	51	1:0.5

In the United States, the average intake of phosphorus is about 1.5 grams a day; the average calcium intake is about 0.7 grams a day. This results in a calcium/phosphorus ratio of 1 to 2. If you consume as little as 400 milligrams of calcium a day, the ratio drops to about 1 to 4.

Adapted from *Nutrition & Health* 1(3): 4, 1979.

The ratio of calcium to phosphorus is also important.

The RDA for phosphorus is the same as for calcium—800 milligrams. Phosphorus is available in many foods, especially protein foods. Cheddar cheese, beef, pork, sardines, tuna, peanut butter, Brazil nuts, cottage cheese, milk, and peas are rich in it.

Calcium utilization can be impaired by an excess of phosphorus. Hence, there is some concern about the high level of phosphorus consumed in soft drinks and meats in the United States.

It is possible for the body to have an excess of calcium (hypercalcemia). Too much vitamin D can increase calcium absorption beyond normal. Some peptic ulcer patients become hypercalcemic after prolonged use of large amounts of milk and antacids. The consequences can include appetite loss and constipation, proceeding to nausea, vomiting, and abdominal pain and, sometimes, muscle weakness, emotional disturbances, confusion, and even psychosis.

Calcium deficiency is much more common. A U.S. Department of Agriculture survey in 1965 found infants, young children, and most men getting the daily requirement of calcium, but almost all women and girls over the age of 8 and many young and adolescent boys and older men were getting inadequate amounts.

A deficiency of phosphorus is rare.

Magnesium

Magnesium once was listed in nutrition books as a trace mineral, needed in only minute amounts. This is no longer the case. In recent years, the Food and Nutrition Board has established an RDA of 350 milligrams for men and 300 milli-

---

There is concern about the high level of phosphorus consumed in soft drinks and meats in the United States.

---

grams for women, which takes it out of the trace mineral class.

Magnesium is now known to be involved in many aspects of body chemistry. It is needed for activating a number of enzyme systems involved in the use of other minerals, some vitamins, and proteins. It is required for both nerve and muscle activity.

Severe deficiency of magnesium is manifested by muscular irritability or twitching, muscle cramps and spasms, weakness, forgetfulness, irritability, depression, mental confusion, and convulsions.

Magnesium is plentiful in seafood, meats, nuts, whole grains, and wheat bran, and it is moderately available in leafy green vegetables, fruits, and dairy foods.

Potassium

Among its many functions, potassium regulates the water content of cells. It participates in the transmission of nerve impulses and the release of energy from carbohydrates, protein, and fats and plays a part in the activity of muscles, including the heart.

Potassium depletion manifests itself by muscle weakness, cramps, diarrhea, vomiting, loss of appetite, apathy, and listlessness and, in severe cases, by irregular heartbeat and heart muscle weakness.

Depletion—which can follow severe diarrhea or the use of certain diuretics for high blood pressure or other purposes—requires the intake of foods rich in potassium and, in some cases, supplementation. Potassium compounds are sold over the counter in health food stores, but self-supplementation is dangerous. Potassium supplements should only be taken at the advice of a physician.

Potassium is widely distributed in foods, especially in meats, milk, vegetables, and fruits. Oranges, tomatoes, and bananas are particularly good sources.

Trace Minerals

Although they are needed only in tiny amounts, trace minerals are essential for health. The importance of some, such

Although they are needed only in tiny amounts, trace minerals are essential for health.

as iodine and iron, has long been recognized. The influence of others has been understood only relatively recently.

Iodine Although needed only in extremely tiny amounts—on the order of 150 micrograms (millionths of a gram) a day—iodine is crucial to the functioning of the thyroid, the small, butterfly-shaped gland in the neck that controls metabolism. Thyroid hormone secretions—less than a teaspoonful a year—are responsible for much of the body's heat production. They help maintain the circulatory system, are needed for muscle health, heighten the sensitivity of nerves, and affect every organ, tissue, and cell of the body. Iodized salt has helped tremendously to solve the problem of iodine deficiency.

Iron Iron is an essential element of hemoglobin, the pigment in red blood cells that transports oxygen from the lungs to all the cells of the body. Inadequate iron intake can lead to anemia, with any or many of a wide variety of symptoms: pallor, weakness, fatigability, irritability, flatulence, vague abdominal pains, neuralgic pains, and heart palpitations. Iron deficiency is common. It can occur as the result of inadequate iron intake and also because of loss of blood (and hence of hemoglobin with its iron content).

According to some estimates, as many as 60 percent of menstruating women in the United States have some degree of iron deficiency.

According to some estimates, as many as 60 percent of menstruating women in the United States have some degree of iron deficiency. Women require more iron than men: the RDA for women is 18 milligrams, for men 10 milligrams. A good diet can help prevent iron deficiency. Meat is a good source of iron; most meats provide 2 to 3 milligrams of iron per 3-ounce serving. Beef liver provides 5 milligrams in a 2-ounce serving, calves' liver is half again as rich in iron as beef liver, and pork liver has twice the iron of calves' liver. An egg contains 1 milligram of iron. Oysters, sardines, and shrimp provide $2\frac{1}{2}$ to 5 milligrams per 3-ounce serving. Most green vegetables provide 1 to 4 milligrams per cup. Other good sources of iron include dry beans, nuts, prunes, dates, and raisins, each containing about 5 milligrams per cup.

Chromium Chromium aids the action of insulin and is essential for the body's proper handling of glucose. The earliest symptom of chromium deficiency is impaired glucose tolerance; chromium deficiency may be related to the onset of diabetes, especially in later life. The estimated maximum need for chromium is only 0.2 milligrams per day. It is found in meats and other animal proteins, whole grains, and brewer's yeast.

Copper A part of many enzyme systems, copper is involved in the normal development of bone and muscle and in the functioning of the nervous system. It is also essential to the formation of hemoglobin from iron. Copper deficiency can cause anemia and may also lead to taste distortion. There is some suspicion that copper deficiency may increase the risk of heart disease. It is estimated by experts that only about 3 milligrams of copper are needed daily. Good sources include shellfish, organ meats, nuts, legumes, and raisins. Excessive amounts are toxic.

Fluorine Not only does fluorine have a role in making teeth more decay-resistant, but there is evidence it may also help to protect against osteoporosis, the bone-thinning and -weakening disease of older people, especially postmenopausal women. Fluorine occurs naturally in some drinking water, but in many communities it is added to fluorine-deficient water.

Manganese Part of many enzyme systems, manganese is needed for normal bone formation, for normal functioning of the nervous system, and for reproduction. In animal studies, a deficiency of manganese has been found to retard growth, impair lactation, and produce seizures. The maximum daily need is estimated to be 5 milligrams. Good sources of manganese include nuts, legumes, whole grains, and tea.

Molybdenum A component of some enzyme systems, molybdenum appears to be involved in the proper utilization of iron. Some iron deficiency anemias unresponsive to iron alone have been corrected with the addition of molybdenum. The maximum estimated daily need of molybdenum is only 0.5 milligrams. Good sources include cereals, legumes, and beef kidney.

Selenium Selenium is believed to protect membranes and other fragile structures from oxygen damage. The maximum estimated daily need is 0.2 milligrams. Grains and onions are good sources of selenium.

Zinc A component of many vital enzymes, zinc is needed for growth and sexual maturation. A deficiency may be related to growth failure, reproductive difficulties, impaired wound healing, some skin disorders, impaired appetite, and abnormalities of taste and smell. The RDA for zinc is 15 milligrams a day for both men and women. Good sources of zinc include seafood, nuts, meat, eggs, and green leafy vegetables.

Avoid Excesses

Although it is important to get adequate amounts of minerals, more is not better and, in fact, can be hazardous. One possible consequence of excessive zinc intake, as mentioned earlier, is copper deficiency. Because zinc supplementation has become increasingly popular, there is increasing scientific scrutiny of this mineral.

After rat studies showed an increase in serum cholesterol in animals fed a high-zinc diet, a human study was car-

> # Although it is important to get adequate amounts of minerals, more is not better and, in fact, can be hazardous.

ried out by investigators of the research and medical departments of the Veterans Administration Hospital and University of New Mexico School of Medicine.

Twelve healthy men with normal cholesterol values received a zinc sulfate capsule twice a day with meals for a 5-week period. The capsules contained 220 milligrams of zinc sulfate—far in excess of the RDA, but a zinc intake not unlike that of some zinc-supplementation enthusiasts.

After 4 weeks, there was a significant decline in blood concentrations of HDL cholesterol, the kind of lipoprotein that is protective against atherosclerosis. By the seventh week, HDL cholesterol levels had fallen 25 percent. Sixteen weeks after the study was initiated, and 11 weeks after the excessive zinc administration was stopped, the HDL cholesterol values returned to near-original levels.

Unquestionably, the best—and safest—way to get the proper amounts of minerals, as well as other nutrients, is from a varied and balanced diet, with supplements used *only* if they are prescribed for a specific purpose by a physician.

Food Additives

More and more foods, from bread to peanut butter to potato chips, have been turning up recently on supermarket shelves in packages marked "No preservatives added," in recognition of the increasing concern, among not only health cultists but also large numbers of citizens, about the safety of chemical additives in foods.

Some of the product changes are somewhat less than rational. Some bread manufacturers have stopped adding the

There is nothing simple about the question of food additives.

mold inhibitor calcium propionate to their products in order to be able to promote them as preservative-free, yet calcium propionate can hardly be considered a hazard. On the contrary, it is safe, incorporates the nutrient calcium, occurs naturally in substantial amounts in Swiss cheese, and stops the growth of molds that may produce toxins.

There is nothing simple about the question of food additives.

The Arguments

Since the 1969 cyclamate ban, additives have had a bad press.

To their defenders, the reaction against additives has worrisome economic, medical, and nutritional implications and is based on false premises. Defenders of additives assert that, for one thing, the idea that foods are free of chemicals except for additives is absurd. Consider, for example, a breakfast of eggs, melon, and coffee. Among other things, it contains such naturally present chemicals as methanol, acetaldehyde, ovomucoid, anisyl propionate, and malic acid.

Defenders also argue that:

* *Many foods, if free of preservatives, may develop hazardous growths—as, for example, the mold (aflotoxins) that may develop on peanuts and on wheat and rye products. Aflotoxins are known to be carcinogenic in animals and are suspected of having some role in human liver cancer.*

* *Many foods naturally contain chemicals which, if consumed in large quantities, can be dangerous. Potatoes, for example, contain solanine, which in excessive amounts can inhibit the functioning of the*

nervous system. Lima beans contain hydrogen cyanide, which can be deadly in excess. But when these chemicals are ingested as part of a balanced, varied diet, they are not harmful.

*　*We know more about the additives to foods than about the chemicals naturally present in foods.*

*　*Additives have kept our food supply plentiful, pleasing, nutritious, and relatively inexpensive; they have reduced food loss due to spoilage, making it possible to enjoy food from many geographic areas; and they have helped to virtually eliminate scurvy, rickets, goiter, and botulism.*

On the other hand, critics of additives reply that while such arguments offer all the favorable factors, they are silent about the dangers. They point to such things as artificial food colorings made from coal tar, indicted long ago for inducing cancer but still used, without ever having been subjected to long-term tests for carcinogenicity. Critics of additives argue that we have had a history in this country of assuming that chemicals added to foods are harmless unless it is proved otherwise, so that cyclamates, for example, were absorbed by consumers for 20 years before being removed from the market.

Critics also are concerned that although many additives may be safe individually, the combination of them—the scores that an individual may consume in a single day—may add up to a hazardous burden, because just how the various chemicals interact is unknown and untested. It should be noted here, however, that possible interactions between chemicals naturally present in foods have had little study either.

Common Additives

There are more than 2000 substances which are added to foods for one or another of four different reasons: to maintain or improve nutritional value, to maintain freshness, to help in processing or preparation, or to make food more appealing.

Nutrients Additives intended to maintain nutritional value, replace nutrients lost in processing, or provide nutrients that may be lacking in the diet include such vitamins as thiamine, riboflavin, and vitamin C. These additives may be found in flour, bread, cereal, rice, beverages, and processed fruit.

Preservatives These include antimicrobials to prevent spoilage from bacteria, molds, and other organisms and to extend shelf life and antioxidants to prevent or delay changes in texture, flavor, or color. Frequently used antimicrobials include vitamin C, citric acid, and calcium propionate. Vitamin C and citric acid also function as antioxidants. Two other frequently used antioxidants are butylated hydroxyanisole (BHA) and butylated hydroxytoluene (BHT). Antioxidants are found in processed foods, baked goods, cereals, snack foods, fats, and oils.

Additives Used to Make Foods More Appealing There are four classes of these: coloring agents, flavoring agents, flavor enhancers, and sweeteners.

Coloring agents are among the most controversial additives because they are used solely for appearance and contribute nothing to nutrition, taste, safety, or ease of processing. There are now thirty-five permitted coloring agents, and they are used in virtually all processed foods. Nearly half are synthetic (now derived from petroleum rather than from coal tar).

In the past 6 years, the Food and Drug Administration has banned four coloring agents from use in foods: a violet

There are more than 2,000 substances which are added to foods for different reasons.

dye used to stamp meats; red dye no. 2, a suspected carcinogen; red dye no. 4, used in maraschino cherries and shown to cause bladder lesions and adrenal gland damage in animals; and carbon black, used in candies. The FDA also proposed to ban orange B, used in sausage and hot dog casings, because of possible contamination with a carcinogen, but the maker voluntarily stopped producing it in 1978.

The two most widely used coloring agents, red dye no. 40 and yellow dye no. 5, are under fire because of possible health risks. Red dye no. 40 is suspected of producing malignant lymph node tumors when fed in large amounts to mice; yellow dye no. 5 causes allergic reactions—mainly rashes and sniffles—in an estimated 50,000 to 90,000 Americans.

Flavoring agents—of which there are some 1700, mostly synthetic—constitute the largest single category of food additives.

If a product contains any added flavoring, natural or synthetic, the label must indicate it. For example, "strawberry yogurt" on a label means all natural strawberry flavor; "strawberry-flavored yogurt" means natural strawberry flavor plus other natural flavorings; "artificially flavored strawberry yogurt" means the product contains only artificial flavorings or a combination of artificial and natural flavorings.

A few flavorings have been prohibited in recent years because of possible health hazards. Safrole, a derivative of sassafras root, once commonly used in root beer, was banned by the FDA after testing indicated it caused liver cancer in rats. Coumarin, often used as an anticoagulant medication, was once present in imitation vanilla extract and other flavorings, but it has been banned from use in food because large amounts could cause hemorrhaging.

Flavor enhancers intensify or modify food flavor without adding any flavor of their own. Some work by briefly inhibiting certain nerves—such as those responsible for bitterness perception—so that perception of other tastes increases.

Among the best known enhancers is monosodium glutamate (MSG), an amino acid, or building block of protein, commonly found in prepared foods and restaurant dishes. Baby food manufacturers who once used MSG in their products stopped doing so voluntarily after studies indicated that large quantities could destroy brain cells in young mice. MSG also produces "Chinese restaurant syndrome"—with such symptoms as headache, chest tightness, and burning sensations—in some sensitive people after consumption of the large amounts often found in Chinese-style foods.

Sweeteners, of course, are commonly used additives. The nutritive types, which are used by the body to produce energy, include natural sugars such as sucrose (table sugar), glucose, and fructose, as well as sugar alcohols such as sorbitol and mannitol. Nonnutritive types, which are not metabolized by the body and so contribute no calories, include cyclamate (currently prohibited) and saccharin.

The addition of sugar to foods is opposed by many on the grounds that it provides only empty calories and contributes to tooth decay, obesity, and other problems.

The sugar alcohols, which are chemical variants of natural sugars, have been promoted as low-calorie alternatives to natural sugars, but they are not actually low in calories. New FDA regulations require manufacturers to indicate that their use in a product does not mean that the product is "low-calorie."

The most widely used sugar alcohol, sorbitol, appears in chewing gum, mints, candies, and dietetic ice cream. Although safe, it can have a laxative effect in large quantities. Mannitol, used in some chewing gums, can cause diarrhea in small amounts.

The nonnutritive sweeteners cyclamate and saccharin have been controversial for a long time. Cyclamate was banned in 1969 on the basis of its causing cancer in animals. Saccharin is under a cloud on the basis of possible health hazards; a Canadian government study showed that it caused bladder tumors in rats.

Additives Used in Preparing and Processing Foods These are the least controversial food additives. There are seven major groups: emulsifiers, stabilizers and thickeners, pH control agents, leavening agents, maturing and bleaching agents, anticaking agents, and humectants.

Emulsifiers are used to allow some liquids to mix which otherwise would not. These compounds keep ice cream and other frozen desserts from separating and in baking serve several purposes, including making batter and dough easier to handle.

Many emulsifiers are of natural origin. Lecithin occurs in milk. Mono- and diglycerides come from vegetables and animal tallow.

One emulsifier which has aroused some concern is brominated vegetable oil (BVO), which is used in citrus-flavored drinks to keep oils in suspension. Residues from this additive are said to accumulate in body fat.

Stabilizers and thickeners, which work by absorbing water, help to keep ice crystals from forming in frozen desserts and prevent evaporation and deterioration of flavor oils used in cakes, puddings, and gelatin mixes. Most are natural carbohydrates such as gelatin (from animal bones and other parts) and pectin (from citrus rind). Vegetable gums (from trees, seaweed, and other plants) are highly effective thickeners, but some, such as tragacanth gum and gum arabic, produce allergic reactions in susceptible persons.

pH control agents affect the safety, taste, or texture of foods by regulating acidity or alkalinity. For example, low-acid canned foods, such as beets, require longer cooking at higher heat than acidic foods if they are to be sterilized; the addition of acids eliminates the need for extra heat which could lower quality. Natural organic acids—such as citric, fumaric, tartaric, and malic acids—are commonly used for canned foods. In some other foods, alkalizers are used to neutralize acids.

Leavening agents, which include yeast, baking soda (sodium bicarbonate), and baking powder (sodium bicarbonate and acid salts), are used to produce carbon dioxide to allow baked goods to rise properly.

Maturing and bleaching agents speed the process by which flour becomes useful for baking—a process which otherwise would require several months of costly storage. Bleaching agents such as benzoyl peroxide also are used to whiten milk for use in some cheeses, such as blue and gorgonzola, known for their whitish curd.

Anticaking agents such as calcium silicate, iron ammonium citrate, and silicon dioxide are used to keep table salt, baking powder, confectioner's sugar, and other powdered food ingredients free-flowing.

Humectants are substances, such as glycerine and sorbitol, which cause moisture to be retained in soft candies, shredded coconut, marshmallows, and other confections.

Practical Answers

The problem of chemicals in our foods—all chemicals, the naturally present as well as the added—is extremely complicated.

The fact is that people have learned by experience, over many millennia, what natural products they can eat with apparent safety—including products now known to contain naturally many chemical substances with potential for toxicity, such as arsenic, lead, cadmium, copper, nitrates, and estrogenic materials. Eating foods with normal levels of these substances has never been known to cause injury, even though some are present at levels closer to known toxic levels than would be allowed today for additives.

Although most of our natural food materials have been accepted as safe on the basis of a long history of use without causing obvious harm, they have never been studied and evaluated scientifically. Therefore there is always the question, recognized by many scientists, about whether any of the natural dietary components such as estrogens, arsenic and cadmium could possibly contribute in any way to degenerative diseases.

It would seem that the best insurance against getting toxic amounts of any single food component is to eat a variety of foods rather than limiting one's diet to a favorite few foods. This would hold for additives as well as for naturally present components.

Additionally, in the case of additives, it makes sense to adopt two guidelines:

* *Minimize as much as possible the use of canned, bottled, or packaged food; rather, concentrate on fresh fruits and vegetables and on foods prepared and cooked at home.*

* *If you must eat canned, bottled, or packaged food, check the ingredients on labels. Avoid those with the longest lists of chemical additives.*

FINDING BETTER FOOD ADDITIVES

A novel technology with promise for the entire field of chemical additives has been developed by Dynapol, a small research concern in Palo Alto, California.

Dynapol apparently has succeeded in attaching food-additive chemicals to molecule chains called polymers, which are too big to pass through the wall of the digestive tract and so are not absorbed. Neither are the food additives.

Upon ingestion, the additives perform their usual intended function and are passed out of the body, rather than absorbed or otherwise retained.

The first polymeric additive that may be marketed, if it is given approval by the Food and Drug Administration, is a preservative with potential as a replacement for chemicals used to retard rancidity in oils, fats, and oil-containing food.

Also in development are a line of nonabsorbable food colorings and a sugar substitute derived from a material extracted from grapefruit rind, called *dihydrochalcone*.

Seven years of research went into development of the non-absorption technology. Along with suitable polymers, it was necessary to find new types of additives with structures compatible with the polymers so the polymers could serve as "sites" for the additives without changing their preserving or coloring properties.

Nonabsorption technology also may have use in the drug and cosmetic fields. One pharmaceutical company is now developing a line of polymeric drugs that will be able to be used to treat digestive tract disorders, such as peptic ulcer and bacterial infections, without the drugs being absorbed and distributed to the rest of the body, where they are not needed.

Health Foods: "Organic" and "Natural"

Upon taking a hard look recently at a product offered as "natural lemon-flavored cream pie," a prominent consumer testing organization discovered that it contains no cream. It does, however, contain sodium propionate, certified food colors, sodium benzoate, and vegetable gum.

That's natural?

"Of course," avowed the also-prominent baker. "Natural," the firm pointed out patiently, modifies "lemon-fla-

The idea that health food is more nutritious than conventional food found in supermarkets, is, in the view of many scientists, fantasy.

vored." The pie contains oil from lemon rinds, so "the lemon flavor comes from natural flavor as opposed to artificial lemon flavor, assuming there is such a thing as artificial lemon flavor."

"Welcome," the testing organization told its subscribers, "to the world of natural foods." It can be a confusing world. It is certainly a controversial one.

Is health food—considered by many to be synonymous with "organic" and "natural" food—more nutritious than the conventional food found in supermarkets? The idea that it is, in the view of many scientists, is fantasy, not fact.

Writing in a Food and Drug Administration publication, an FDA Bureau of Foods dietician and nutritionist, Marilyn Stephenson, put it this way:

> Advocates of "health," "organic," and "natural" foods—terms for which there is little agreement as to their exact meaning—frequently proclaim that such products are safer and more nutritious than conventionally grown and marketed foods. Although most of these claims are not supported by scientific evidence, it is difficult for the public to evaluate truth from fancy—particularly in regard to use of the term "natural" for everything from whole grain flour or bread to potato chips. Claims or suggestions that certain health foods or diets prevent or cure disease or provide other special health benefits are, for the most part, folklore, and sometimes fabrication.

Health food enthusiasts respond that eating food untouched by additives and preservatives and grown without herbicides, pesticides, and manufactured fertilizers makes sense.

If it does make sense, it is at a price. Health food products sell at a premium; the prices are sometimes staggering, as in the case of a 1-pound loaf of whole wheat bread, which may cost almost twice as much in a health food store as in a supermarket.

According to an article by Myron Winick, M.D., in *Medical World News*, there is nothing objectionable in health foods aside from cost and the need for greater care in preservation, "so long as people are not duped by the health food industry into expecting advantages that are not there. If they want to pay more for the possibility that this is more healthful, fine."

BEYOND REGULATION

Many consumers do not know that the First Amendment to the Constitution of the United States places some kinds of statements about food and nutrition beyond the reach of federal regulation through its protection of free speech and free press.

If the label on a food product makes false or misleading claims, the FDA can take action on the grounds that the product is mislabeled or misbranded. If false claims are made in ads or in other materials directly promoting the product, the Federal Trade Commission may be able to take action.

But the labels on or promotions for fad foods or diets often do not make any direct claims that can be shown to be false. Instead, they refer to a book, a pamphlet, a speech, or a magazine article that has praised the product. Thus, these indirect promotions receive the protection of the First Amendment.

Scientific rebuttal of food and nutrition myths published and perpetuated in faddish literature often is futile. As Dr. Edward H. Rynearson, recently retired from the Mayo Clinic, has said, "Americans love hogwash." We have fables that natural vitamins are superior to synthetic vitamins, that the soil in this country is "all worn out," or that the use of organic fertilizers results in better crops than manufactured fertilizers. And we have many minor myths: that organic (fertilized) eggs are nutritiously superior to infertile eggs, that raw milk is better than pasteurized, and the like.

The terms *organic, natural,* and *health* are so loosely and often interchangeably used that they are difficult to define—so much so that the FDA has taken no position on their use in food labeling.

FDA Consumer, HEW Publication (FDA) 79-2108, July 8, 1978

It would seem, however, that in the health food industry, as in any other, what is offered is not always what it is claimed to be.

Organic—What Does It Mean?

In chemistry, the word *organic* refers to compounds containing carbon in their molecules—a vast array of them, ranging from animal and plant products to petrochemicals and pesticides.

Organic as applied to health foods, however, means foods grown without use of pesticides, synthetic fertilizers, and other chemicals, relying instead on natural fertilizers such as manure and compost.

How Much Difference Does Organic Growth Make?

If there is any difference between the nutrient content of plants grown organically and of those grown with the help of chemicals, it has yet to be scientifically established.

Dr. Emil M. Mrak, a renowned authority on agriculture, has pointed to scientific experiments conducted for 25 years at Cornell University and elsewhere in this country and in England, which have found no differences between organic foods and those treated with manufactured fertilizers. It appears that once removed from the garden, organically grown foods cannot be distinguished from those that have been commercially fertilized.

Plants produce some of their own nutrients and derive

It appears that once removed from the garden, organically grown foods cannot be distinguished from those that have been commercially fertilized.

others from the soil through their roots. Regardless of the source, roots absorb nutrients in inorganic form, and any organic matter has to be broken down by soil bacteria to release inorganic elements before there can be absorption. Since only the nutrients themselves are absorbed, plants are not concerned about the nature of the source. As far as plants are concerned, needed nutrients can come from any fertilizer, synthetic or natural.

If a soil is known to be deficient in a particular mineral, the mineral can be incorporated in a synthetic fertilizer or it may be obtainable from the decomposition of organic wastes.

Organic wastes—natural fertilizers—are not necessarily perfect fertilizers. Manure, for example, has plentiful phosphate but much less nitrogen, which may not be ideal for some plants. Manure also may contain pests, such as insects, worms, and disease-carrying bacteria.

Free of Pesticides?

A claimed advantage of organically grown foods is the absence of pesticides, which, supposedly, should make the produce free of pesticide traces or residues. But, as an FDA Consumer Report has pointed out:

> The fact is that many of these foods do contain pesticide residues. Even if no pesticides are used on a particular crop, some chemical residues often remain in the soil for years after the last application of a pesticide on a previous crop. In addition, fresh residues may be deposited from drifting sprays and dusts or from rainfall runoff from nearby farms. Traces of pesticides may be found in both organic and conventional foods, but these residues normally are within federal tolerance levels, which are set low enough to protect the consumers.

Tests by various agencies and laboratories of organic-labeled foods purchased from health food stores and comparable nonorganic foods bought at supermarkets have shown little difference in pesticide-residue levels.

For example, in 1972, the New York State Department of Agriculture and Markets analyzed 55 food products labeled "organically grown" and found that 30 percent contained pesticide residues. At the time, the department was sampling about 2000 nonorganic foods annually and finding pesticide residues in about 20 percent.

In 1978, an analysis by Wayne State University and Michigan State University investigators of five brands of bread from health food stores and five from supermarkets showed that all ten had traces of pesticide residues.

In 1979, when KNXT-TV in Los Angeles was doing a series of programs on organic foods, it had a Los Angeles laboratory—one that does pesticide testing for both government agencies and private companies—test twenty-eight samples of fruits and vegetables from health food stores, labeled "organically grown," and fourteen samples of similar nonorganic produce from supermarkets. The laboratory could find no overall difference in pesticide levels. Only two samples contained no residues at all, and one of those was from a supermarket.

Also in 1979, in connection with a *New West* magazine article, another California laboratory that tests for pesticides for the U.S. Department of the Interior analyzed organic lettuce from six San Francisco health food stores and nonorganic lettuce from a supermarket. It found pesticide residues in five of the six organic lettuces as well as in the supermarket lettuce. The supermarket lettuce contained 0.01 parts per million of phosdrin, an aphid-killing spray, but the tests also found six times that much in one and eight times as much in another organic lettuce. A third organic lettuce also contained residues of phosdrin and two other pesticides.

FERTILIZER: AN OVERVIEW

"Two hundred years ago, the average family in the Western world had to spend most of its time grubbing a meager living from the soil. The lack of fertilizer, the presence of pests that diminished crops, and the absence of knowledge about plant breeding all combined to keep most people hungry. Then chemists discovered that plants were actually nourished by inorganic chemicals. Phosphate, potash, nitrate, and ammonia were needed. They could come either from the breakdown of manure by soil bacteria or from rock phosphate, inorganic potash, nitrates, and ammonia salts. The agricultural revolution was on. Farmers became able to feed more and more city folk.

"A century ago, farmers were helpless against the fungus blight which turned their potatoes into a black slime. As a result, one million people starved to death during the Irish potato famine. Pesticides to control the blight were not yet available.

"As agricultural knowledge increased by leaps and bounds, farming became increasingly scientific. Plant and animal breeding gave us fine new strains of grains, vegetables, fruits, poultry, pigs, and cattle. More efficient fertilizers and a wide variety of pesticides were developed. Rare delicacies became commonplace.

"The new chemical methods required careful regulation to see that farmers used them properly. Pure food laws were passed to make sure that only insignificant traces of unwanted pesticide residues were present in foods. These laws appear to be working well. There has not been one case of illness in America which can be attributed to a scientific agricultural procedure. In contrast, in countries where "organic" fertilizers (such as human waste) are used, food poisoning from disease organisms is quite common."

Thomas H. Jukes, Ph.D., University of California at Berkeley, and Stephen Barrett, M.D., Lehigh Valley Committee against Health Fraud, Inc., in *The Health Robbers*, Stephen Barrett, M.D., and Gilda Knight (eds.), George F. Stickley Co., Philadelphia, 1976.

"The Best Protection"

Says an FDA report:

> Since chemically and organically grown foods do not differ in looks, taste, or chemical analysis, the only way to assure that a product labeled as "organically grown" is truthfully labeled would be to keep watch over the product from planting to harvest to sale, and to check soil and water reports. Such a program, of course, would be prohibitively expensive.
>
> The possibility for fraud is apparent when the consumer doesn't know if the storekeeper is honest, when the storekeeper can't tell if the distributor is honest, and when the distributor doesn't know if his suppliers are living up to their

promises. Because of this and the premium prices placed on organic foods, it's not surprising that conventional foods at times have been substituted for organic foods. . . .

It would be inaccurate to imply that all elements of the health food industry engage in shady marketing practices. Some distributors and growers supply affidavits or certificates for foods grown and handled according to "organic and natural" precepts. Many health food operators truly believe in health foods and are sincere in trying to provide consumers the "real" thing.

Reading the labels and trusting in the health food store manager appear to be the best protection for the consumer interested in purchasing these foods. Recently it was reported that a natural food store in California removed all vitamins, which are high profit items, from its shelves. The management had learned that most of a product labeled "Rose Hips Vitamin C from Natural Sources" was synthetic. Unable to confirm that similar practices do not occur in other natural vitamin supplements, the store stopped handling vitamins and suggested that people get them from a pharmacy where the pills aren't labeled as natural and they're cheaper.

That's excellent advice from both a scientific and economic viewpoint. Vitamins from natural sources have no nutritional superiority over synthetic vitamins, and the Food and Drug Administration prohibits such claims in food labeling.

NATURAL VERSUS SYNTHETIC VITAMINS

This claim that [natural vitamins are better than synthetic ones] is a flat lie and anyone who makes it should be immediately classified by you as a quack. Each vitamin is a chain of atoms strung together as a molecule. Molecules made in "factories" of nature are identical to those made in the factories of chemical companies.

Victor D. Herbert, M.D., Hematology and Nutrition Laboratory, Bronx Veterans Administration Hospital

IF YOU NEED ADVICE

There are many unbiased sources of sound nutritional information where you live or to whom you can write. Most large medical centers have qualified nutritionists or dieticians. Many of the former are members of the Society of Nutrition Education, the American Institute of Nutrition, or the American Association of Clinical Nutrition. Many dieticians are members of

Molecules made in "factories" of nature are identical to those made in the factories of chemical companies.

the American Dietetic Association.

If there is no one to consult near you, send a stamped, self-addressed envelope to Virginia Bayles, Membership Secretary-Treasurer, Consulting Nutritionists, 5018 Indigo, Houston, Texas 77096. In New York, you can write Consulting Nutritionists in Private Practice, P.O. Box 345, Cold Spring, New York 10516, or call (212) 582-2800.

You can also contact local chapters of the American Heart Association or the American Diabetes Association, or write to the U.S. Department of Agriculture, Office of Governmental and Public Affairs, Washington, D.C. 20250.

There are newsletters available in libraries or by subscription, such as *Nutrition and Health*, Columbia University College of Physicians and Surgeons, 701 West 168 Street, New York, New York 10032, and *Environmental Nutrition*, 52 Riverside Drive, Suite 15-A, New York, New York 10024.

Adapted from *The New York Times*, March 25, 1981, p. C19.

Natural—What Does It Mean?

Natural, as applied to foods, is supposed to mean that the products contain no preservatives or artificial additives and have undergone minimal processing. Certainly, there is nothing undesirable in that.

But beware.

A Federal Trade Commission staff report issued in 1978 told of nationally advertised cereals and processed frozen foods labeled "natural" that contained chemical preservatives. Some foods labeled "natural" also contain heavy amounts of added salt and sugar, the report noted. It went on to add: "The term 'natural' has been applied to foods which run the gamut on extent of processing."

Once largely limited to health food stores, products labeled "natural" today are flowing in ever-increasing quantities onto supermarket shelves.

Is Natural Food Better?

Some may be. Minimal processing in some cases leaves foods more nutritious.

But judiciously used processing is hardly without benefits. Pasteurization of milk, which kills potentially dangerous microorganisms, is not to be dismissed lightly. In some cases, frozen foods can be more nutritious than fresh foods, which lose nutrients if not consumed promptly.

If there are questionable additives, there are also many serving highly useful purposes: calcium propionate retards the growth of mildew in bread and contributes calcium to the diet as well, and sorbic acid avoids potentially harmful mold growth in cheese.

Do "natural" potato chips deserve to be considered any less of a "junk " food than conventional potato chips? They may come at a premium price, without preservatives, cut from unpeeled potatoes, and sometimes with sea salt instead of regular "table" salt (no demonstrated advantage). But both come from potatoes, are loaded with salt, and are prepared in such a way that they are high in calories as well.

You can buy natural granola-type cereals with added oil, but they have more fat, usually more sugar, and considerably more calories than conventional cereals.

What Passes for Natural

A recent survey in *Consumer Reports* has turned up an interesting series of examples of questionable application of the word *natural* to food products.

Consumer Reports points, for instance, to two 15-ounce cans of tomato sauce, available side by side in one store. One sauce claimed on its label to have "no citric acid, no sugars, no preservatives, no artificial colors or flavors." There were no such ingredients in the other sauce either, a house brand, "but their absence was hardly worth noting on the label, since canned tomato sauce almost never contains artificial colors or flavors and doesn't need preservatives after being heated in the canning process." There was one clear difference between the two products: price. The house brand was selling for 29 cents, the other for 85 cents.

Some other examples:

✱ *A brand of "natural chocolate-flavored chocolate chip cookies" with fine print on the label indicating the cookies contain both artificial flavor and the chemical antioxidant BHA.*

* *A "whole grain date-filled fruit and oatmeal bar" whose label proclaimed "naturally good flavor" but whose ingredients include "artificial flavor."*

* *A well-known brand of crackers red-labeled as a natural product with no preservatives, but with an ingredient list including calcium propionate "to retard spoilage."*

* *A well-known brand of "high-protein cereal" which implies that it is "natural" through much material on the package about "nature," with that word used four times and the word "natural" once but never to describe the product inside, which, among other things, contains artificial color and BHA.*

* *The increasing presence of the claim "no artificial preservatives" on labels of jars of jam and jelly—as if this has not always been true, since sugar is all the preservative needed for such products.*

* *A prominent brand of so-called natural margarine, which, in fact, has been highly processed from its original vegetable oil state.*

Regulation

Some effort is beginning to be made to assure that when the word *natural* is used, it has some meaning.

In 1980, Maine put into effect a law which requires that for any product with the label "natural" to be sold in the state, it must have had only minimal processing and contain no preservatives, additives, or refined additions such as white flour or refined sugar.

In an effort to end confusion, the Federal Trade Commission recently proposed the first federal standard governing the advertising of natural foods.

According to the FTC definition, a food may be advertised as being natural if it contains no artificial ingredients and has no more processing than it would generally get in a home kitchen:

Under the definition, minimal processing includes such things as washing or peeling fruits and vegetables; homo-

> ## Some effort is being made to assure that when the word *natural* is used, it has some meaning.

genizing milk; canning, bottling, and freezing foods; baking bread; aging meats; and grinding nuts. It does not include such steps as chemical bleaching of foods.

The commission standard also allows use of the word *natural* in advertisements if deviations from the standard are spelled out. For example, an ad could say: "Natural but contains bleached flour."

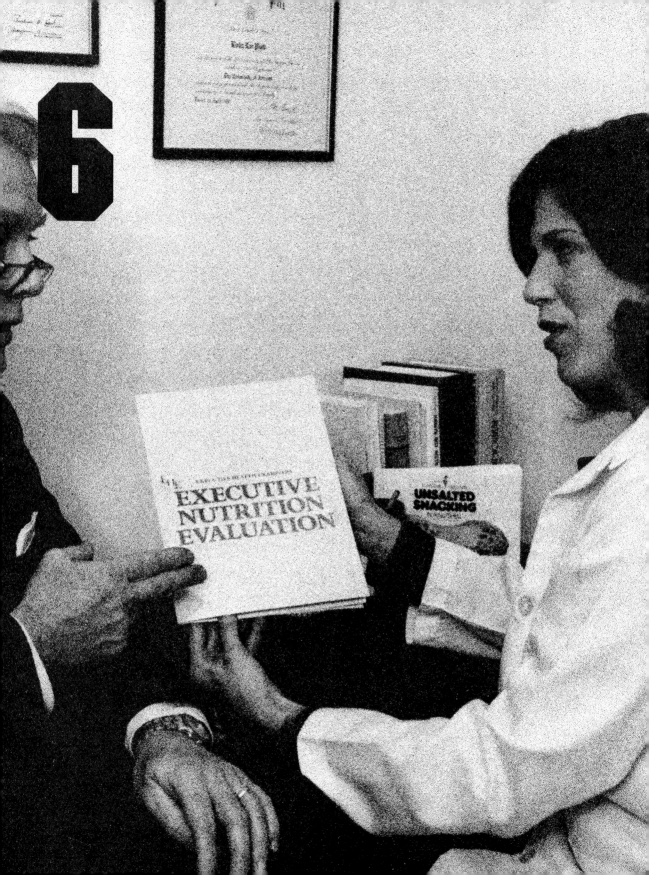

OTHER NUTRITIONAL CONSIDERATIONS

Dietary fiber *has become a nutritional buzzword. It has been endowed by some with a near-magical aura, although there is much confusion about what it actually is.*

Alcohol—long considered unmitigatedly bad from the health standpoint—has recently earned some striking credits in its favor.

Caffeine—in coffee, tea, and much else—has been making news, sometimes confusing news.

So, too, the link between diet and cancer.

And vegetarianism—*no longer dismissible as faddist indulgence—has tripled its adherents in a generation.*

This chapter examines all of these.

Dietary Fiber

Dietary fiber is, very literally, the indigestible part of food. You eat it—and excrete it.

It was largely ignored until recently by nutritionists, who are used to thinking in terms of digestion of foods and the subsequent absorption and use by the body of nutrients.

Now supermarket shelves are stocked with a variety of new "high-fiber" foods. More than a dozen cereals directed at adults contain the word *bran* in their names or mention fiber prominently on the front of the box.

When the Surgeon General's Report on Health Promotion and Disease Prevention called for efforts to produce a "public health revolution," one recommendation was more consumption by Americans of foods rich in fiber—whole grains, cereals, fruits, and vegetables.

Shortly afterward, in testimony before the U.S. Senate's Nutrition Subcommittee, Arthur Upton, M.D., then director of the National Cancer Institute, also urged "generous" intake of dietary fiber as a measure that might help reduce the risk of one of our most common and deadly malignancies, cancer of the colon.

The New Interest

Fiber itself is nothing new. Our grandparents called it "bulk" and "roughage," and until relatively recently it was very much a part of the ordinary diet.

About the turn of the century, however, the invention of

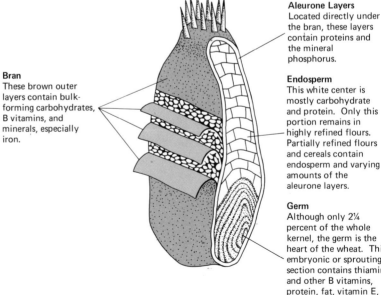

Bran
These brown outer layers contain bulk-forming carbohydrates, B vitamins, and minerals, especially iron.

Aleurone Layers
Located directly under the bran, these layers contain proteins and the mineral phosphorus.

Endosperm
This white center is mostly carbohydrate and protein. Only this portion remains in highly refined flours. Partially refined flours and cereals contain endosperm and varying amounts of the aleurone layers.

Germ
Although only 2¼ percent of the whole kernel, the germ is the heart of the wheat. This embryonic or sprouting section contains thiamin and other B vitamins, protein, fat, vitamin E, minerals, and carbohydrates.

Kernel of wheat

modern roller mills made it possible economically to re-move the outer husk of cereal grain kernels, and with it the fiber, to produce refined white flour. Quickly thereafter, fiber intake plummeted—to the point where, until quite recently, cereal fiber intake in the United States and much of western industrialized society stood at only one-tenth of what it used to be.

Even as fiber consumption was falling markedly, the inci-dence of many diseases was shooting up. Appendicitis, for example, became noticeably common only in the twentieth century; coronary heart disease was considered rare 50 years ago.

Yet nothing comparable was occurring among rural Afri-cans living, as they always had, on their native unrefined diets. They certainly were subject to infections; they some-times went hungry; but eating unrefined cereal as a staple, getting about 25 grams (almost an ounce) of fiber daily—many times as much as the average westerner—they rarely experienced the chronic western diseases.

Only recently was any of this recognized—as the result of the epidemiologic detective work of a group of British physicians led by Denis Burkitt, a surgeon famed for his dis-covery and cure of a childhood cancer named after him (Burkitt's lymphoma). Many of these men, including Burkitt, had worked for years as mission and government physicians in Africa. For years they, too, were unaware of the possible significance of the local diet. Then, gradually, they were struck by a series of facts.

Although cancer of the colon has become a scourge of western nations, ranking as the second most common cause of cancer death after lung cancer, it is rare in east Africa. In the United States it now strikes 100,000 persons a year, but in Kampala, Uganda, the rate is only one-fifteenth as great. Annually, 300,000 American appendixes are removed, but in African villagers, appendicitis is virtually nonexistent. Diver-ticulitis (abnormal outpouchings of the colon that can cause severe pain and may require surgery) is present in over one-third of Americans and other westerners over the age of 40. Dr. Burkitt reported that in 20 years in Africa he had not seen a single case.

Moreover, as some Africans moved from native villages to

cities and adopted western low-fiber diets, the incidence of western diseases began to rise sharply. At one hospital in Uganda, for example, the appendectomy rate increased more than 20 times between 1952 and 1969. In 1956 came the first case of coronary heart disease reported in east Africa—in a 48-year-old high court judge who had lived for 20 years on a western diet.

AN OLD CONCERN: OVER-PROCESSED FOODS

Contrary to common belief, the concern about overprocessed food is not a twentieth-century revelation.

Hippocrates, the father of medicine, recommended eating unbolted wheatmeal bread (made from flour still containing bran) for its "salutary effects upon the bowels."

In the nineteenth century, Sylvester Graham (called by some the father of food reform in the United States) claimed that indigestion was caused by too refined a diet, and that putting bran back in wheat flour would correct it. Even today, his name has been immortalized in that common staple, the graham cracker.

The physician attending Graham at his death was Dr. J. H. Kellogg, who later, in 1895, introduced the first ready-to-eat cereal to our nation in the form of toasted wheat flakes.

Peter G. Lindner, M.D., *Obesity/Bariatric Medicine* 7(4):134, 1978.

How Fiber Works

Fiber adds bulk. Upon reaching the intestinal tract, it absorbs water and swells. That leads to bulkier but soft, well-formed stools, and that in turn prevents constipation, with its characteristically small, hard, pebbly, slow-moving stools.

Native African stools weigh as much as four times those of westerners, and transit time—the interval between a meal being eaten and the remains being excreted—averages only 35 hours for African villagers, compared to 90 hours for many westerners.

Constipation—extremely common in westerners but rare in rural Africans—is more than a nuisance. It leads to straining, which may be responsible for a series of problems. It has been proposed that straining raises pressure in the colon, which may cause the outpouchings of the colon wall in diverticular disease. With straining, pressure within the abdomen also rises and may cause the stomach to push up through the diaphragm, producing hiatus hernia, with its possible heartburn, regurgitation of stomach acid back up into the esophagus, and burning pain in back of the breastbone.

Raised pressure in the abdomen can be transmitted elsewhere—to the leg veins and to the veins in the anal region—and so, it has been proposed, such pressure from constipation-induced straining may be responsible for varicose veins and hemorrhoids (which are also varicose, or unnaturally swollen, veins).

Evidence is accumulating that restoring fiber to the diet can achieve some highly desirable effects. In one study, for example, the substitution of two slices of fiber-rich wholemeal bread and the addition of 2 teaspoonfuls of fiber-rich bran daily led, within 3 weeks, to marked increases in stool weight and speedup of transit time, with an end to constipation. There have been reports as well of relief for hemorrhoid sufferers as stools soften and straining is eliminated.

Until quite recently, fiber, or roughage, was banned for people with diverticular disease in the mistaken belief that it was too irritating. Now there have been many reports that adding fiber to the diet produces striking improvement. In one large study, 88.6 percent of patients improved, and many who had been scheduled for surgery no longer required it.

Other Possible Benefits

In addition to such benefits as overcoming constipation and helping in diverticular disease, dietary fiber may have other benefits. The evidence for this comes from varied studies—some from direct human research, others from animal experimentation. Some are epidemiologic, attempting to relate various disease statistics to local dietary customs. Still other projected benefits are based on what are essentially theoretical hypotheses, taking into account both the physical characteristics of foods and physiology.

Dietary fiber may provide protection from cancer of the colon and rectum.

Cancer of the Colon Epidemiologic studies of various populations, comparing disease incidence with dietary fiber intake, have suggested that dietary fiber may provide protection from cancer of the colon and rectum.

To account for the protection, the following hypothesis has been offered: Cancer of the colon and rectum results from cancer-causing chemicals (carcinogens) produced by bacteria in the bowels. When stools are small, hard, and slow-moving, the bacteria in them have more time to act and the carcinogens they produce are more concentrated in the stools, are retained longer, and thus can act for longer periods on the lining of the colon.

Some investigators suggest, the extra water, bile acids, salts, and fat bound by added fiber may serve as solvents to remove many chemical factors that might be carcinogenic.

It has also been suggested that a high-fiber diet may alter the types and numbers of bacteria in the bowel and possibly inhibit their production of carcinogens. One study, which supports this possibility, showed that one class of microorganisms that produce compounds convertible to carcinogens is present in western stools in much greater amounts than in stools from populations in underdeveloped countries.

Although fiber may well be protective against cancer of the colon, many investigators caution that more definitive evidence is needed. Theories based on epidemiologic findings may be misleading. For example, some recent studies indicate that the incidence of colon cancer in various areas correlates even better with the amount of fat in the diet than with the amount of fiber.

Heart and Blood Vessel Disease Fiber may help reduce elevated cholesterol levels, which are believed to be involved in atherosclerotic artery disease, heart attacks, and strokes.

In one study, for example, fiber-rich rolled oats reduced cholesterol levels in 3 weeks. In another, when high-fat diets were fed to healthy men, their cholesterol levels shot up; when one form of fiber, chickpea, was added to these diets, cholesterol increase was inhibited. In other studies, guar gum and pectin—other forms of fiber—have reduced cholesterol levels. Bran, however, does not appear to change blood cholesterol levels.

Diabetes In one of the first studies of the possible effects of fiber on diabetes, a decline in insulin requirements was noted in patients who ate increased amounts of fiber-rich foods. Another found blood glucose levels of patients taking insulin to be significantly higher on a low-fiber than on a high-fiber diet. Since then, several other preliminary studies have shown a drop in blood glucose levels and in the need for insulin (or for oral antidiabetes drugs) after the institution of high-complex-carbohydrate and high-fiber diets—in some patients within a few weeks. Diabetic patients should have the advice of a physician before changing to this diet.

Gallstones Stones in the gallbladder may form from excess cholesterol in the bile. Recent studies suggest that a fiber rich diet reduces bile cholesterol. A study at the Univeristy of Bristol, England, found bile cholesterol reduced in 80 percent of patients.

Weight loss Preliminary investigations indicate that a high-fiber diet may help promote weight loss, and further studies are certainly indicated.

At the University of Bristol, Kenneth Heaton, M.D., a pioneer fiber investigator, noted that when he, his wife, and several colleagues increased fiber in their diets by eating wholemeal bread instead of refined white bread, they lost weight—not dramatically, but gradually and smoothly. The losses went as high as 15 pounds—and without any attention to calories or attempts to restrict the amount eaten.

Wholemeal breads, pound for pound, frequently contain

fewer calories than conventional white breads, and they may also reduce food consumption because they increase the feeling of satiation.

In a study in Denmark, twenty-five healthy nurses took a little less than 1 ounce (24 grams) of wheat bran a day for 5 weeks. Their food intake remained constant, yet they lost weight. One possibility is that fiber, by shortening transit time through the intestines, may decrease absorption of nutrients.

Fiber—More than Just a Single Substance

For a long time, all fiber was considered to be "crude fiber," which is what is left after a food sample is treated in the laboratory with a solvent, hot acid, and hot alkali. Chemically inert, this residue consists mostly of the lignin and cellulose in the food being analyzed.

Dietary fiber is different, however. It is defined as including all the components of a food that are not broken down in the digestive tract to produce small compounds which can be absorbed into the bloodstream.

Dietary fiber includes hemicelluloses, pectic substances, gums, mucilages, and other carbohydrates, as well as lignin and cellulose. These compounds occur mainly in the cell walls of plant tissue, and their total greatly exceeds the total of crude fiber.

The various fiber components have different properties and effects; thus, the fiber composition of food is significant in discussing its effect on the body. For example, pectin, lignin, guar gum, oat hulls, and barley have been found to have some cholesterol-lowering effect, but bran and cellulose have none.

Food Sources of Dietary Fiber

Many varied foods supply significant amounts of dietary fiber and its components. As the Institute of Food Technologists points out, the total dietary fiber in both fresh vegetables and fruits may appear to be relatively low, but that is because of their high water content. The fiber actually represents a substantial proportion of the solids content.

HIGH-AND LOW-FIBER MENUS

Low-fiber and high-fat	*High-fiber and low-fat*
BREAKFAST	
Instant powdered orange drink	1 orange
1 slice white bread	1 slice whole wheat bread
1 tsp butter	1 tbsp apple butter
6 oz whole milk	6 oz skim milk
$\frac{1}{2}$ cup canned peaches	1 tbsp almonds and 1 tbsp raisins
1 cup cornflakes	1 cup 40% bran flakes
SNACK	
10 potato chips	$1\frac{1}{2}$ cup popcorn (plain)
12 oz carbonated beverage	12 oz apple juice
LUNCH	
3 oz roast beef on white bread	3 oz turkey (white meat) on whole wheat
$1\frac{1}{2}$ tbsp mayonnaise	bread, mustard and lettuce
20 french fries	Tossed salad with lemon juice
6 oz instant onion soup	1 cup vegetable soup
Cola	8 oz apricot nectar
Gelatin dessert and topping	1 apple, medium
SNACK	
Snack pie	$\frac{1}{2}$ cup dried fruit and nut mix
Coffee and cream	6 oz vegetable juice
DINNER	
4 oz fried chicken	4 oz broiled fish
$\frac{1}{2}$ cup macaroni and cheese	1 cup gumbo (corn, tomatoes, okra)
$\frac{1}{4}$ cup cole slaw	1 cup brown rice
$\frac{1}{2}$ cup buttered peas	1 cup fresh relish (radishes, celery,
2 dinner rolls	green peppers, carrot curls)
2 tsp butter	1 slice banana bran bread*
$\frac{3}{4}$ cup ice cream	$\frac{1}{4}$ cantaloupe wedge
TOTAL	
45 g fat	27 g fat
4.7 g fiber	17.23 g fiber

* *Banana bran bread:*

$\frac{1}{2}$ cup butter or margarine	$\frac{3}{4}$ cup sugar
2 eggs	$1\frac{1}{2}$ cup mashed ripe bananas
1 tsp vanilla	1 cup bran
$1\frac{1}{2}$ cup unsifted all-purpose flour	$\frac{1}{2}$ tsp baking soda
2 tsp baking powder	$\frac{1}{2}$ tsp salt

Mix in large bowl: margarine, sugar, eggs, bananas, and vanilla.
Add bran and let stand for 5 minutes.
Mix dry ingredients together and blend with banana mixture.
Bake in greased, floured, 9 by 5 by 3 inch loaf pan at 350°F for 70 minutes.
When done, cool for 10 minutes; then remove from pan and cool on rack.
SOURCE: *Nutrition & Health* 1(5):5–6, 1979.

TOTAL DIETARY FIBER AND COMPOSITION IN SOME FRUITS, VEGETABLES, AND WHEAT PRODUCTS

Food	Total dietary fiber (fresh basis), g/100 g (3½ oz)	Composition of the dietary fiber, %		Composition of the noncellulosic fraction, %			
		Polysaccharides, noncellulosic	Cellulose	Lignin	Hexoses	Pentoses	Uronic acids
Cabbage, cooked	2.83	37	63	Trace	16	55	28
Carrots, cooked	3.70	60	40	Trace	20	35	45
Peas, frozen, raw	7.75	69	27	2	48	22	30
Tomato, raw	1.40	47	32	21	14	42	44
Apple, flesh only	1.42	66	33	<1	20	35	40
Banana	1.75	64	21	15	54	19	27
Pear, flesh only	2.44	54	28	19	20	46	35
Plum, raw, flesh and skin	1.52	65	15	19	28	46	25
Strawberry, raw	2.12	46	16	38	22	33	45
White flour (72%)	3.45	80	19	1	80	11	9
Brown flour (95%)	8.70	72	18	10	44	45	11
Wholemeal flour	11.00	72	20	8	39	48	13
Bran	48.00	74	18	7	19	60	12

SOURCE: Adapted from tables published in the Marabou Symposium on Food and Fiber.

Potatoes and starchy vegetables supply significant amounts of fiber if eaten in fairly large quantities. The lignin content of most vegetables is low, while that of fruits is highest in those containing lignified seeds, such as the strawberry, or lignified cells in the flesh, such as the pear. The noncellulosic polysaccharides in these foods are usually rich in pectic substances (uronic acids) and in pentoses.

Use of wholemeal flour instead of white flour increases the lignin in the diet and provides as well a threefold increase in total dietary fiber from that source.

What is a Good High-Fiber Diet?

Fiber is bran and bran is fiber—or so it seems to many. But that is not the case at all.

Certainly, wheat bran—composed of the outer layers of wheat, which are removed in the preparation of white flour

A COMPARISON OF CRUDE FIBER AND DIETARY FIBER IN CERTAIN FOODS

Food	Crude fiber,* g/100 g (3½ oz)	Dietary fiber,† g/100 g (3½ oz)
Breads and cereals:		
White bread	0.2	2.72
Whole wheat bread	1.6	8.50
All-bran cereal	7.8	26.70
Cornflakes	0.7	11.00
Puffed wheat	2.0	15.41
Puffed wheat, sugar-coated	0.9	6.08
Vegetables:		
Broccoli tops, boiled	1.5	4.10
Lettuce, raw	0.6	1.53
Carrots, boiled	1.0	3.70
Peas, canned	2.3	6.28
Sweet corn, cooked	0.7	4.74
Fruits:		
Apples, without skin	0.6	1.42
Peaches, with skin	0.6	2.28
Strawberries, raw	1.3	2.12
Nuts:		
Brazil nuts	3.1	7.73
Peanuts	1.9	9.30
Peanut butter	1.9	7.55

* Data from U.S.D.A. Handbook 8, *Composition of Foods.*
† Data from David Southgate, Medical Research Council, Cambridge, England.

—is a rich source of fiber. It can be bought as miller's bran —preferably as coarse flakes, rather than fine, because it is more effective in the coarse form. Two tablespoons provide about 7 grams, or ¼ ounce, of dietary fiber, which is usually adequate to benefit bowel behavior.

However, there are other sources of fiber, and to get maximum benefit from dietary fiber and its various components selections should be made from a variety of whole-grain products, fruits, and vegetables, including:

* *Cereals such as old-fashioned, slow-cooking (not instant) oatmeal; shredded wheat; cereals labeled as being all-bran or largely made up of bran.*

* Breads and other bakery products made with wholemeal flour (whole wheat or whole rye).

* Seeds, including whole sesame seeds and sunflower seeds, and seed-filled berries such as raspberries and blackberries.

* Other fruits and vegetables, such as mangoes, carrots, apples, brussels sprouts, eggplant, spring cabbage, corn, oranges, pears, green beans, lettuce, winter cabbage, peas, onions, celery, cucumbers, broad beans, tomatoes, broccoli, cauliflower, bananas, rhubarb, potatoes, turnips.

Can You Have Too Much Fiber?

There is a tendency when some important nutritional finding is reported as the result of research, for it to be applied to an extreme. Eating as much as 10 tablespoons of bran a day has been urged in some popular regimens—with no evidence whatever that such large amounts are necessary or valuable. In fact, a sudden, excessive increase in the amount of fiber eaten can cause painful intestinal bloating and diarrhea. It is even possible that very large amounts of fiber could cause enlargement and twisting of the colon.

It has been suggested that too much of the pectin form of fiber may cause decreased absorption of vitamin B_{12}. There is also a possibility that excessive fiber intake could lead to loss of minerals such as zinc, iron, calcium, copper, and magnesium because of the binding of these minerals by phytic acid, which is present in some plant-based foods.

Fiber is not a panacea. It is one part—an important part—of a properly balanced diet.

Our Recommendations

Fiber is not a panacea. It is one part—an important part—of a properly balanced diet. Fiber research is still relatively young. At this point, there are no definitive answers to questions of how much and what kind of fiber is ideal. What clearly makes sense are moderation in amounts of fiber eaten and diversity in the sources.

Alcohol

Alcohol—its use is two-pronged.

Does it relax tension? It may, but it can also impair reason and judgment. Does it heighten sexual desire? Perhaps it does, but it can have the opposite effect on performance.

Clearly, alcohol in excess can be hazardous to one's health, even deadly. It is toxic to many body tissues. Now, however, there is evidence that it may be, in moderation, a life extender through an apparently beneficial effect on the heart.

New Evidence: Alcohol and Heart Attacks

Recent research findings from epidemiologic, or population, studies and from clinical and laboratory studies suggest that alcohol in moderate amounts is associated with fewer heart attacks, possibly because it reduces the formation of fatty deposits inside the coronary arteries supplying the heart muscle. Several epidemiologic studies have shown that moderate drinkers are less likely to die from heart attacks than are abstainers. Clinical studies using coronary arteriography (special x-ray techniques for examining the coronary arteries) have reported that heavy alcohol users have relatively low plaque buildup in their arteries. Autopsy studies, too, have found that heavy drinkers generally tend to show little atherosclerosis. Their deaths are usually from other diseases or other causes, such as accidents.

There has been other suggestive evidence, as well, from cross-cultural studies that moderate alcohol consumption may be beneficial. Countries such as Spain, Portugal, France, and Italy, which have relatively high per capita rates of alcohol consumption, have comparatively low death rates from coronary heart disease.

Further confirmation has come from a large-scale California study.

The California Findings

Recently, Arthur L. Klatsky, M.D., of the Kaiser Foundation Hospital in Oakland, California, reported the results of a massive study at Kaiser-Permanente system facilities throughout northern California. He and fellow investigators analyzed the hospitalization of 87,926 adults, between 1971

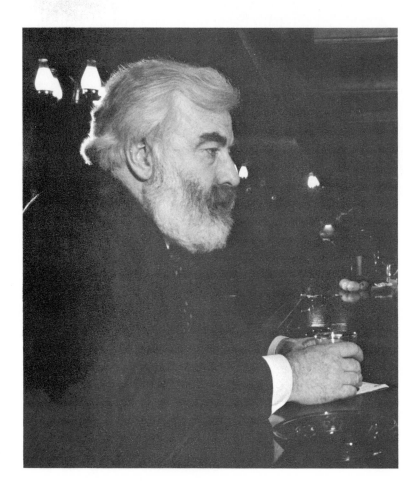

and 1976, whose drinking patterns had been recorded routinely a decade earlier. Since 2105 had reported taking six or more drinks a day, the investigating team selected three comparison groups of the same number—abstainers, persons taking no more than two drinks a day, and those taking three to five drinks regularly. All together, the study covered more than 8000 adults.

It was not surprising at all when the heaviest drinkers turned out to be the likeliest to be hospitalized for accidents, cirrhosis of the liver, other digestive diseases, alcoholism, and mental disorders, as well as for cancer, respiratory problems, high blood pressure, and stroke.

But it was surprising when the people with the fewest hospitalizations proved to be not the abstainers but those taking one or two drinks daily.

When it came to hospitalization rates for coronary heart disease and heart attacks, they were significantly higher among nondrinkers. Of nondrinkers, 8 percent were hospitalized for coronary disease, compared with 5.9 percent of less-than-two-a-day drinkers.

What Does Alcohol Do?

Alcohol appears to increase the level of protective high-density lipoproteins (HDLs) in the blood.

At the Arteriosclerosis Research Center at Wake Forest University, Thomas Clarkson, M.D., has recently carried out studies with monkeys which indicate that the severity of coronary artery atherosclerosis, as it developed in animals fed a high cholesterol diet with or without alcohol, was largely determined by the inclusion or exclusion of alcohol.

Alcohol appears to increase the level of protective high-density lipoproteins (HDLs) in the blood.

Alcohol increased HDL concentration. It also decreased the molecular weight of low-density lipoproteins (LDLs). Heavier LDLs in the blood were found to be strongly associated with atherosclerosis in the animal studies.

Still more evidence of alcohol's beneficial effects on HDL levels has come recently from human studies. A particularly noteworthy one was carried out by W. Willett, M.D., and a group of investigators in the Department of Preventive Medicine at Harvard Medical School and in the Framingham Heart Study.

Aware that physical activity, body weight, and other variables may affect HDL levels, the investigators wanted to determine whether alcohol itself could be responsible for increasing HDL or whether in fact the benefits attributed to alcohol might have been due to activity and other variables.

Using a study group of ninety male physicians, 29 to 60 years of age, who had participated in the 1979 Doctors' Marathon, they measured HDL levels and correlated the results with each man's quantitative alcohol intake.

By well-established statistical procedures (multiple regression analysis), the investigators were able to assess independently the effects of alcohol, physical activity, weight, and other variables. They found that the level of HDL was higher in those men whose rate of alcohol consumption was higher. The statistical analyses showed that alcohol itself, not the physical activity, caused the elevated HDL levels, even though each of the subjects was a marathon runner.

Drawbacks

If moderate use of alcohol may offer some benefit, it is important to put this in perspective. It has been established that alcohol in excess is harmful. Ten million adult Americans—7 percent of those 18 years old or older—are estimated to be alcoholics or problem drinkers. According to the 1979 U.S. Surgeon General's Report, *Healthy People,* "Of all adults who drink, more than a third have been classified as either current or potential problem drinkers, with women making up one-fourth to one-third of the latter."

Weight control is also a consideration. A.J., a 50-year-old advertising account executive was not considered an alcoholic, yet a routine annual examination at Executive Health Examiners revealed abnormal liver enzymes. Further tests showed that his liver was normal, but the EHE physician referred A.J. to the nutritionist for counseling about weight control because he had been gaining weight rapidly and was 70 pounds above the ideal weight for his height.

Discussion about his diet disclosed an excessively high daily intake of alcohol—several cocktails plus wine at lunch and dinner. The large amount of alcohol he drank was definitely contributing to his weight problem and was probably responsible for his abnormal liver enzyme test as well.

A number of counseling sessions, utilizing such techniques as role playing, record keeping, and drink compromises and substitutions were required to help him modify his drinking pattern. Eventually, he lost half of his excess weight and cut his alcohol intake by two-thirds, and his liver enzymes returned to normal.

The Surgeon General's Report underscores these facts:

* *Alcohol misuse is a factor is more than 10 percent of all deaths in the United States, about 200,000 a year.*

* *It is associated with half of all traffic deaths.*

* *Cirrhosis, which ranks among the ten leading causes of death, is largely attributable to alcohol consumption. (We should add that the liver, the only body organ which can metabolize alcohol, is a main target for other alcohol damage. When forced to use alcohol as an energy source, instead of fatty acids, which are its normal source, the liver becomes fatty as the fatty acids accumulate there. Alcoholic hepatitis, a liver inflammation, may be triggered by heavy drinking bouts. Also an alcohol-damaged liver may be unable to detoxify poisons and carcinogens that get into the body.)*

* *Alcohol use is associated with cancer, particularly of the liver, esophagus, and mouth. Primary liver cancer—malignancy originating in the liver—is often attributed to alcohol consumption. People who drink and also smoke cigarettes have an ever greater risk of developing esophageal cancer.*

✱ *Excessive drinking during pregnancy can produce infants with severe abnormalities, including mental retardation.*

It has also been established by many studies that the heart is not immune to damaging effects from excessive alcohol, which can damage heart muscle cells and reduce the heart's pumping efficiency. It can raise the blood level of triglycerides, the fatty materials that can play a role in artery clogging. Heavy drinkers commonly suffer from cardiomyopathy (a heart muscle disorder), high blood pressure, and abnormal heart rhythms, and many alcohol abusers die of cardiovascular disorders at relatively early ages.

ALCOHOL NOW: SOME AUTHORITATIVE VIEWS

"Most emphatically, alcohol is not the public health measure to use for reducing coronary heart disease risk. On the other hand, it is important to recognize the role of alcohol in the natural history of coronary heart disease."

Tavia Gordon, consultant to the National Heart, Lung and Blood Institute

"To jump to the conclusion that abstainers or infrequent users should be encouraged to drink is premature. Given the present state of knowledge, it is prudent to try to reduce other well-documented risk factors for coronary heart disease—such as stopping smoking, increasing physical activity, eating less salt and animal fats and maintaining body weight."

Charles Kaelber, M.D., National Institute of Alcohol Abuse and Alcoholism

"The data are not yet definitive enough to allow physicians to advocate alcohol as a therapeutic means of raising HDL-C levels. Nevertheless, the old family doctor who prescribed *spiritus frumenti* for mood elevation of the aging patient may have been unwittingly ahead of his time. In the future, physicians may well find themselves prescribing the "four Rs": rest, relaxation, running, and rum."

Hospital Practice, January 1981.

"A simplistic view of alcohol as good or not good for the heart is not appropriate. I don't think drinking should be one of the mainstays of heart attack prevention. . . . Obviously you can't tell a person who's quit because of alcohol problems to begin again. But drinking is not dangerous for most people, and one or two a day may be protective."

Arthur L. Klatsky, M.D., Kaiser-Permanente Medical Center

What Do You Do?

Clearly, the recent findings about possible benefits from moderate alcohol intake in terms of heart disease are encouraging—to a point—and for some, but not all, people.

What is moderate intake?

Pending further studies of what might constitute an ideal intake for the heart without other risk, it appears to be about two bottles of beer, or two 4-ounce glasses of wine, or 2 ounces of whiskey daily. At least, for now, this seems to be the level at which, for most healthy people, benefits may outweigh risks.

For people with certain medical problems, however,

Americans say they drink only about half as much alcohol as they apparently consume, according to Charles Kaelber, M.D., of the National Institute of Alcohol Abuse and Alcoholism.

Reporting to a recent symposium on alcohol and cardiovascular disease, Dr. Kaelber noted that in national surveys respondents report drinking an average of about $\frac{1}{2}$ ounce of alcohol per day. Yet beverage sales data reveal that they actually purchase the equivalent of nearly a full ounce per person per day.

The credibility of an individual's self-report probably decreases as his or her alcohol intake increases, according to Kaelber. As drinking approaches problem levels, "the desire as well as the ability to be an accurate self-reporter may diminish," he reported.

"These biases complicate investigations of the association between alcohol use and various cardiovascular diseases since so much reliance currently must be placed on self reports to assess a person's alcohol consumption."

AMERICANS UNDERREPORT THEIR DRINKING BY HALF!

CALORIC CONTENT OF ALCOHOLIC AND CARBONATED BEVERAGES

	Calories*
Beer (4.5% alcohol by volume, 3.6% by weight), 12 oz	144
Gin, rum, vodka, whiskey (bourbon, rye, scotch):	
86 proof (36.0% alcohol by weight), 1½ oz (1 jigger)	107
100 proof (42.5% alcohol by weight), 1½ oz (1 jigger)	127
Mixed drinks:	
Creme de menthe, ⅔ oz	67
Daiquiri, 3½ oz	122
Highball, 8 oz	166
Manhattan, 3½ oz	164
Martini, 3½ oz	140
Old-fashioned, 4 oz	179
Tom Collins, 10 oz	180
Wines:	
Dessert (18.8% alcohol by volume, 15.3% by weight), 3½ oz	137
Table (12.2% alcohol by volume, 9.9% by weight), 3½ oz	85
Champagne, 4 oz	84
Sherry, 2 oz	84
Carbonated beverages, nonalcoholic:	
Carbonated waters:	
Sweetened (quinine sodas), 10 oz	88
Unsweetened (club soda), 10 oz	0
Tom Collins mixer, 10 oz	130
Ginger ale, 7 oz	62
Root beer:	
12 oz	140
10 oz	117
Cola type:	
12 oz	133
10 oz	111
"Pop" (fruit-flavored sodas, 10–13% sugar):	
12 oz	158
10 oz	130
Diet cola and pop:†	
12 oz	72
10 oz	60

* *Calorie* is used here as it is commonly used in discussions of nutrition; each "calorie" is actually equivalent to 1 kilocalorie (kcal), or 1000 calories.
† Food and Drug Administration regulations (January 1970) allow diet cola and pop to contain a maximum of 6 calories per fluid ounce.
SOURCE: *A Maximal Approach to the Dietary Treatment of the Hyperlipidemias*, Subcommittee on Diet and Hyperlipidemia, Council on Arteriosclerosis, American Heart Association, 1973.

even moderate levels of alcohol may be too much, and abstinence in some cases may be best. These problems include, of course, alcohol-related conditions such as fatty liver and cirrhosis. They also include epilepsy and diabetes. And it goes without saying that continued abstinence may be best for anyone who has had to give up drinking before because of problem drinking or alcoholism.

Caffeine

Americans are hardly in a class with Voltaire, a king of coffee lovers, who drank more than 50 cups a day. But we do well enough as consumers of the brew, averaging about 16 pounds worth per person per year and drinking up to half of the world production.

We also take in huge amounts of caffeine in addition to what we get in coffee. Most people know there is caffeine in coffee and tea, but not as many realize it is also present in some soft drinks. Even fewer may know that they are consuming caffeine when they sip a cup of cocoa, munch on a chocolate bar, or take some pills for a headache or cold. It is even used in some foods.

Coffee: Friend or Enemy?

For a time, not so long ago, a cloud hung over coffee. One of the first reports suggesting a possible association between coffee and coronary heart disease appeared in 1963 to the consternation of lovers of the beverage.

To make matters worse, in 1972 and again in 1973 came

Much of the cloud over coffee has lifted.

other reports suggesting that people who drink more than 5 cups a day have about twice as great a risk of having a heart attack as people who do not drink coffee.

In 1974 there were sighs of relief when two important studies were published contradicting the findings of the earlier ones.

One was an analysis of health checkup questionnaires which had been completed by 197 men, 40 to 79 years of age, some time before they died suddenly. Comparison with data on other men of comparable age and characteristics obtained from 250,000 computerized health checkup questionnaires revealed no significant increase in the incidence of sudden death from heart attacks among those who drank even more than 6 cups of coffee a day.

The other report came from the Framingham Heart Study in which, over a 12-year period, careful records of daily coffee consumption were kept for the thousands of participating men and women. No significant differences could be found between coffee drinkers and non-coffee drinkers for onset of coronary heart disease or development of such heart disease indications as chest pain (angina pectoris) or heart attacks.

The Framingham report also found no significant relationship between coffee consumption and development of stroke and other heart and blood vessel problems not related to coronary heart disease. The data also showed no significant effect on high blood pressure or blood cholesterol levels, although this had been suggested in some earlier studies.

More recently, because smoking had been shown to adversely affect blood cholesterol levels and there remained some belief that coffee might do the same, Siegfried Heyden, M.D., and other investigators at Duke University Medical Center carried out a study of 361 people. As we noted earlier, high LDL cholesterol levels can be harmful, and the Duke study found LDL levels to be significantly higher among those who smoked and consumed 5 or more cups of coffee daily than among nonsmokers who abstained from coffee. However, although smoking and coffee drinking interacted to increase LDL levels and total blood cholesterol, coffee drinking alone had no apparent effect on cholesterol.

Other Caffeine Effects

Caffeine, which qualifies as a drug, has several effects on the body. It acts as a diuretic, promoting urination, and as a stimulant for the central nervous system. Although it does not affect everyone in the same way, if consumed in large enough doses, it can cause insomnia, nervousness, irritability, anxiety, and disturbances of heart rate and rhythm.

Some people, whether they realize it or not, become addicted to the stimulant effect of caffeine and may experience withdrawal symptoms—typically, headache—when they do not get their usual amount.

Ulcers? Caffeine in coffee and other drinks does tend to stimulate stomach acid secretion. The stimulation appears to be mild and transitory in healthy people but may be sustained in those with ulcers, suggesting that ulcer-disposed people may be more sensitive to caffeine and should moderate their intake.

At various times, caffeine has been suspected of being linked to other diseases, such as diabetes and bladder cancer—but to date no firm evidence has been found to prove a cause-and-effect relationship.

J.V., a 23-year-old secretary who came to Executive Health Examiners at the suggestion of her supervisor, had no idea of what caffeine and a poor diet were doing to her.

Her boss, who was a vice president of a manufacturing concern, recognized that J.V. ate very little, substituting coffee, cola drinks, candy bars, and cigarettes for food. He suggested that perhaps this was why she had become irritable, lacked energy, and complained of an upset stomach.

J.V. was surprised at what the records of her food intake revealed. She had no idea how much caffeine she was consuming in the form of cola drinks, coffee, and candy bars, how much sugar she was getting, and how little "real" food she was eating.

Gradually, this pattern was changed. Because J.V. lived alone and disliked cooking, the nutritionist suggested that she purchase some high-quality convenience food, eat more fiber, and get "coverage" so she could take advantage of the daily hot-meal special at the company cafeteria. Within a few months, J.V. reported that she felt "like a new person."

A SOBERING FACT: COFFEE AND HANGOVERS DON'T MIX

Coffee, thought by many to counteract the effects of alcohol, may in fact postpone your recovery from a hangover.

In a hangover state, you are really recovering from the direct toxic effect of alcohol, reports James Dexter, M.D., a researcher into alcohol effects.

Large amounts of alcohol dilate blood vessels, disrupt metabolism, alter dream-state sleep, and dehydrate the body—four totally separate effects with different recovery periods. What is more, the first three of these effects can, in susceptible people, trigger a migraine headache,—which is a greater discomfort than what most people experience with a hangover.

To speed the body's return to normal, Dexter recommends taking in fluids and carbohydrate calories in the form of fruit juice. People with moderate to severe hangovers need a liter of fluids immediately on waking to counteract the body's dehydration, and over the next 24 hours they need to drink another liter more than they normally would.

People commonly underestimate the extent of dehydration, and some compound the problem by drinking large amounts of coffee, which acts as a diuretic, further adding to the dehydration.

Since an alcohol-irritated stomach may keep a person from eating, Dexter suggests a forced-fluid regimen of fruit juices to counteract the double whammy of dehydration and stomach irritation.

Still, as Dexter notes, the body needs time before blood vessels return to normal and before disrupted sleep is recovered.

"If in a night you normally have an hour of REM (rapid eye movement, or dream-state) sleep," says Dexter, "during high levels of alcohol you would have maybe 10 minutes of REM. Then the next night you would recover the loss by having nearly two hours of REM sleep."

This sleep recovery phenomenon, when accompanied by an adequate amount of food and fluids, signals the end of the hangover, Dr. Dexter reports reassuringly.

Caffeinism Syndrome

In sensitive people, large amounts of caffeine can produce a syndrome, or set of symptoms, mimicking the psychiatric disorder of chronic anxiety. While tranquilizers and other drugs then may be used, the need is not for new drugs but simply for a reduction in the intake of caffeine.

Among the symptoms of the caffeinism syndrome are restlessness, irritability, insomnia, headache, muscle twitching, racing pulse, flushing, lethargy, nausea, vomiting, diarrhea, and chest pain.

Individual sensitivity varies. For some people 250 milligrams of caffeine a day may be enough to provoke a reaction. That amount is considered sizeable, yet many people exceed it almost daily. For example, if you drink 3 cups of coffee and a cola and take two caffeine-containing headache tablets, your total intake of caffeine is about 500 milligrams.

Caffeinism was first brought to light at an American Psychiatric Association meeting several years ago by John Greden, M.D. Greden noted several dramatic cases of people who had benefited when their caffeine problem was recognized and their caffeine intake was reduced.

One, a young nurse married to an army physician, sought help because of a 3-week siege of lightheadedness, tremulousness, breathlessness, headache, and irregular heartbeat. When nothing physically wrong could be found, she was referred for psychiatric help with a diagnosis of anxiety reaction.

She refused to accept the diagnosis. In fact, she was the first to suspect a possible dietary cause, linking her symptoms to a marked increase in her coffee consumption. She had started making coffee by a new method and finding the result superior, had taken to drinking 10 to 12 cups a day, containing a total of more than 1000 milligrams of caffeine.

Her symptoms disappeared within 36 hours after she stopped drinking coffee. She was later challenged with caffeine twice, with the symptoms returning each time and disappearing again when the caffeine was eliminated.

Another case involved a 37-year-old military officer referred for psychiatric help after a 2-year history of chronic anxiety. His almost-daily symptoms included dizziness, tremulousness, apprehensiveness about job performance, restlessness, frequent diarrhea, and persistent sleep problems.

He drank 8 to 14 cups of coffee a day, often drank hot cocoa at bedtime, and liked only cola soft drinks, of which he drank three or four a day. He was incredulous at first that caffeinism might be the reason for his problems; he was also unwilling to try cutting down his caffeine intake, but he finally gave in. A few weeks later, he reported marked improvement.

The Final Word

For some people—those very sensitive to its effects—caffeine, obviously, is best avoided. But for many, if not most, people, caffeine—in moderation—has its value. Coffee, for example, smells good, tastes good, and produces mild eu-

THE CONFUSION ABOUT CAFFEINE INTAKE

There is no easy way to tell how much caffeine you may consume in coffee, tea, cocoa, soft drinks, and other caffeine-containing products. Studies and tests often add to the confusion, because the same standards are not always followed.

Some studies are based on a manufacturer's directions for brewing a cup of coffee or tea. In the home, some brew it strong; others brew it weak. Some brew it for a long time; others, a short time. It is also not easy to compare one study with another because cup sizes are not always the same.

At the request of the National Coffee Association, biochemist Dr. Alan W. Burg reviewed the scientific literature on coffee and caffeine content and, noting the discrepancies, suggested that the 150-milliliter cup (5 ounces) be considered the average size for research.

Basing his data on twenty-nine coffee and thirteen tea products, he suggested that there was an *average* of 85 milligrams of caffeine in a 5-ounce cup of percolated, roasted, ground coffee, 60 milligrams in instant coffee, 3 milligrams in decaffeinated coffee, and an average of 30 milligrams in instant tea. He also found a range of 64 to 124 milligrams of caffeine in percolated coffee, 40 to 108 milligrams in instant coffee, 2 to 5 milligrams in decaffeinated coffee, 42 milligrams (based on one sample tested) in bagged tea, 30 to 48 milligrams in leaf tea, and 24 to 131 milligrams in instant tea.

Compare this with the findings of the Addiction Research Foundation of Ontario, which did a caffeine study based on forty-six home-brewed coffee samples and thirty-seven tea samples, some of which had cream and other dilutants in the sample. Cup sizes also varied.

The Foundation's findings were that percolated coffee contained 39 to 168 milligrams of caffeine to a cup, with 74 milligrams as a median; drip or filtered coffee 56 to 117 milligrams, with 112 milligrams as a median; decaffeinated coffee 1 to 2 milligrams; and tea 8 to 91 milligrams, with 27 milligrams as a median.

Other studies have found 12-ounce cola type soft drinks to contain 32 to 65 milligrams of caffeine; cocoa, from 5 to 40 milligrams; a $\frac{1}{2}$-ounce chocolate bar, 10 milligrams; a headache tablet, 65 milligrams; and some stay-awake tablets, up to 100 milligrams.

Soft drinks, including the cola type that contain caffeine, are the number one beverage of Americans today, with coffee number two. According to beverage industry sources, an American consumes an average of 33.6 gallons of soft drinks each year. The average consumption of coffee is 27.8 gallons per person each year, followed by milk, at 24.8 gallons per person.

Adapted from *FDA Consumer*, October 1980.

phoria, reduced fatigue, and increased alertness. Tea lovers and appreciators of other caffeine-containing beverages may feel the same about their favorites.

For most people, moderation is the key. Avoiding excess, they can enjoy these pleasures with little, if any, likelihood of harm.

Cancer and Diet

Salt may aggravate high blood pressure. Sugar has been implicated in diabetes. Beef and butter—saturated fats—are linked to coronary heart disease and heart attacks.

What about food and cancer?

For years, investigators at the National Cancer Institute and elsewhere have been studying the possible relationship between dietary influences and cancer, particularly of the digestive tract. They have looked with suspicion, too, at the

CAFFEINE CONTENT OF FOODS AND DRUGS

Coffee (6 oz):
Automatic drip	181 mg
Automatic perk	125 mg
Instant	54 mg

Tea (6 oz):
Iced tea	69 mg
Red Rose	45 mg (weak), 62 mg (medium), 90 mg (strong)
Tetley	18 mg (weak), 48 mg (medium), 70 mg (strong)
English breakfast	26 mg (weak), 78 mg (medium), 107 mg (strong)

Soft drinks (12 oz):
Mountain Dew	54 mg
Mellow Yellow	51 mg
Dr. Pepper	38 mg
Pepsi-Cola	38 mg
Coca-Cola	33 mg
Tab	32 mg
RC Cola	26 mg

Cocoa:
Chocolate candy (2 oz)	45 mg
Baking chocolate (1 oz)	45 mg
South American (5 oz)	42 mg
Milk chocolate candy (2 oz)	12 mg
African (6 oz)	5 mg

Drugs:
Dexatrim capsules (Thompson)	200 mg/tablet
Nodōz tablets (Bristol-Myers)	100 mg/tablet
Anacin (Whitehall)	32.5 mg/tablet
Midol (Glenbrook)	32.4 mg/tablet
Coricidin (Schering)	30 mg/tablet

SOURCE: *The Health Effects of Caffeine*, American Council on Science and Health, March 1981.

possible relation of fats in the diet to breast cancer development.

Even though the precise link between diet and cancer remains far from clear-cut, it has been reported by some authorities that dietary factors appear to be responsible for 50 percent of all cancers in women and 20 percent of all cancers in men. Although debated, some estimates have gone higher—up to 60 percent of all cancers in women and 40 percent of those occurring in men.

The Clues

The strongest indications of a link between diet and cancer come from epidemiologic studies of population groups.

In many western countries, colon cancer has become the most common malignant condition other than skin cancer in both men and women, and its incidence is rising.

Incidence rates vary greatly, however. Barring death from another cause, men in Connecticut, for example, have 1 chance in 30 of developing cancer by age 74; in Colombia the rate is 1 in 300; in Nigeria, 1 in 700.

The highest rates occur in countries with the highest consumption of beef, which is rich in animal fats. This includes the United States, Scotland, New Zealand, Canada, and Denmark. It also includes the beef-eating countries Argentina and Uruguay, setting them apart from other South American populations, where colon cancer rates are generally low. Colon cancer incidence is highest in New Zealand, where per capita beef consumption is even higher than in the United States.

The relation between fats and colon cancer is underscored by changes in bowel cancer incidence in groups whose dietary habits are altered through migration. The Japanese, for example, with a diet traditionally low in fat, have less than a third of the American incidence of bowel cancer, but Japanese-Americans, who have adopted the western habit of eating large amounts of beef and butter, run much the same bowel cancer risk as other Americans.

On the other hand, colon cancer rates are low for Seventh-Day Adventists, who are vegetarian and whose diet has 25 percent less fat and 50 percent more fiber than the average U.S. diet. Proportionately increased colon cancer rates occur among those Adventists who deviate from vegetarianism.

The Bowel Cancer Mechanism—Does Fiber Help?

Precisely how fat contributes to colon cancer is not yet clear. One theory is that fats increase concentration of bile acids in the large bowel and also stimulate the growth of certain intestinal bacteria. These bacteria may then act on the bile acids to produce carcinogens.

There is evidence to support this theory. Populations with high colon cancer rates have increased fecal bile acids. High correlations are also found between colon cancer death rates and the concentrations of a colonic bacterial product.

Some investigators believe that a high-fiber diet helps to protect against colon cancer by absorbing or diluting the carcinogens. Belief in the value of fiber is based on the observation that colon cancer is either unknown or very rare among primitive or developing populations whose diets have a very high fiber content. Recent additional epidemiologic reports support the belief. A collaborative study in Denmark and Finland, for example, has shown that the Finns, who consume foods high in both fat and fiber, have a relatively low rate of bowel cancer. Copenhagen people, with a fourfold higher risk of colon cancer, eat only one-half the dietary fiber of people in the low-risk area of Finland.

Dietary Fat and Breast Cancer

Breast cancer risks also vary with the fat content of the diet. As far back as 1966, one study found a highly significant correlation between breast cancer rates and fat consumption in twenty-four different countries; the higher the fat intake, the higher the breast malignancy risk. Another, later study of diet and many other variables found the highest correlation among all variables, including all foods studied, to be for breast cancer death rates and total dietary fat.

Japanese women brought up in the United States on an American diet have the same incidence of breast cancer as their American Caucasian counterparts, but the rate in Japan is only one-fifth that among American women. However, within Japan itself, dietary habits are changing. Recently the overall fat intake there has increased 2.5 times and animal protein intake has increased nearly 2 times. Breast cancer mortality rates in Japan have also begun to rise.

In the United States, women vegetarians have a much lower breast cancer rate than do other women, apparently as a result of eating far less or no animal fat and meat.

How fat influences the development of breast cancer is unknown. One theory is that fat affects the balance of female hormones.

Stomach Cancer

There may be something positive to the American diet that has led to a marked drop in the incidence of stomach cancer. In the United States 50 years ago, the stomach cancer rate was 30 per 100,000 men and 22 per 100,000 women; currently the U.S. rate is down to 7.5 and 3.7, respectively. These changes suggest some dietary factor.

Around the world today, there is marked variation in incidence rates, with high-risk areas such as Japan, Iceland, Chile, and Finland suffering five or more times greater rates than low-risk areas such as the United States, New Zealand, and Australia.

No single food has yet been identified that is common to all the high-risk populations, but some food–stomach cancer correlations have been reported. For example, increased risk in Japan has been shown in relation to pickled vegetables and dried salted fish. Among Japanese migrants to Hawaii, lower risk has been associated with the use of western-type vegetables, notably lettuce and celery.

Nitrosamines are powerful carcinogens. They result from the interaction of nitrates and nitrites with other substances in food. Nitrosamines rapidly produce stomach cancers in over 80 percent of laboratory animals, even in species in which the natural occurrence of such cancers is virtually unknown.

In the past, nitrites—which can enter into nitrosamine formation in the stomach by combining with constituents of protein foods—were added to meats, fish, and pickled vegetables in quantities as high as 5000 parts per million to improve color and flavor and help protect against botulism. Currently, in the United States, lower levels, up to only 150 parts per million, are being used, and these levels may decline to only 10 parts per million soon after processing.

Vitamin C can inhibit the formation of nitrosamines from nitrites, and some investigators believe that the reduction in stomach cancer among Americans may be due, at least in part, to increased consumption of fruits and green leafy vegetables containing vitamin C.

The way people cook food has been studied recently by investigators interested in the possible relationship of cancer to diet. Preliminary studies show that populations with a high intake of charcoal-broiled meat or fish may be at higher risk of genetic mutation, and some studies have implicated frying or broiling in the development of some cancers.

What to Do

Like heart disease, cancer involves many risk factors, ranging from heredity—about which you can do nothing—to diet —about which you *can* do something.

Until much more information is made available by research, this is the best dietary advice: Use common sense. Take in fewer calories overall and less fat in particular, especially saturated fat, and see that your diet includes reasonable amounts of fiber and plentiful amounts of fresh fruits and vegetables.

Cancer involves many risk factors ranging from heredity—about which you can do nothing—to diet—about which you *can* do something.

With interest in the relationship between diet and cancer intensifying, research is intensifying too.

Vitamin A and related compounds, which together are classified as retinoids, are now known to be active in cell differentiation, the process by which young new cells acquire the characteristics of the tissue for which they are destined. Cancer-producing agents arrest that differentiation.

There is laboratory evidence that retinoids may enhance the normal processes of differentiation blocked by carcinogens. For example, in laboratory cultures of tissues from the air passages, cells develop abnormally in the absence of retinoids. Addition of retinoids reverses the process. In animal studies, retinoids have been found to reduce the incidence of cancer induced by chemical carcinogens.

In a Norwegian study with a large group of men, thirty-six developed lung cancers over a 5-year period. In those with a high vitamin A intake, the cancer incidence was reduced by as much as 80 percent compared with those with a low vitamin A intake.

In Japan, where much of the dietary intake of retinoids comes from yellow-green vegetables, a study involving 280,000 persons over a 10-year period found that among smokers a daily intake of yellow-green vegetables was associated with a 20 to 30 percent reduction in lung cancer incidence. Among ex-smokers, the cancer risk reduction was much greater, suggesting that retinoids may play a role in the recovery process.

Natural retinoids have limited use. They tend to be highly toxic because they are deposited excessively in the liver. Retinoids have been artificially produced with the hope of reducing such problems. One of the most promising, 13-*cis*-retinoic acid, appears not to be deposited and stored in the liver and seems better able to reach body sites where it is needed. Not available for general use, it is now under experimental investigation and shows some promise in counteracting chemically induced cancer in laboratory animals.

On the basis of research to date, it would seem, as one investigator has put it, that "no human population at risk for the development of cancer should be allowed to remain in a vitamin A deficient state," which underscores the importance of a well-rounded diet, including the intake of yellow-green vegetables.

Some green vegetables, it now appears, have a protective effect beyond that associated with vitamin A. Broccoli, cabbage, brussels sprouts, and cauliflower recently have been found to inhibit chemically induced breast and stomach cancer.

Some trace elements are also under study. Selenium, for example, when given at the rate of 2 parts per million of the daily diet to laboratory animals, appears to inhibit the formation of both chemically induced and spontaneous tumors. Some population studies also seem to indicate a protective effect for selenium, particularly against colon, rectal, breast, and ovarian cancer.

Among foods rich in selenium are whole wheat bread and flour, oat and wheat cereals, brown rice, lobster tail, cod, flounder, oysters, beef liver and kidney, fresh garlic, and mushrooms.

Vegetarianism

Vegetarianism is no longer looked upon as a faddish way of eating. For those who follow it, it can be an alternative way of eating a healthy diet.

Currently an estimated 7 million Americans—three times as many as just a generation ago—consider themselves vegetarians. Some avoid meat simply because it is too expensive, some believe it is wrong to kill animals for food, and for others it is a religious matter not to eat meat.

In 1974, when the National Research Council of the National Academy of Sciences evaluated vegetarian diets, it found that all but the most restricted are nutritionally safe. "The most important safeguard for average vegetarian con-

Vegetarianism can be an alternative way of eating a healthy diet.

sumers," its report declared, "is great variety in the diet"—a safeguard equally applicable to meat eaters.

What Vegetarians Eat

Vegans, vegetarians who eat no animal products in any form, are relatively rare in the United States. Those who do eat dairy products and eggs are known as *lactovovegetarians*, and those who eat milk products but no eggs are known as *lactovegetarians*.

Lactovovegetarians have access to all four basic food groups: dairy products (milk, cheese, yogurt, ice cream, and other dairy products); vegetables and fruit; grain products (bread, pasta, cereals, rice and other grains); and protein sources (eggs, dried beans and peas, peanut butter, lentils, soybeans, nuts, and seeds). Although lactovegetarians do not use eggs, there are protein-rich foods in the meat group that they can eat, and protein can be found in the other food groups.

For lacto- and lactovovegetarians, the greater the diversity of vegetables, fruits, cereals, legumes, nuts, and seeds added to the dairy products in the diet, the better the nourishment. They can improve the quality of protein by combining dairy products with grain products—for example, cereal with milk, and macaroni with cheese.

Vegans need to select foods with great care to get adequate nutrients, with special attention to protein. Only proteins from animal muscle, milk, and eggs contain the amino acids needed for protein synthesis in the body in approximately the proportions the body needs. Proteins from vegetables, grains, and nuts provide significant amounts of many amino acids, but they do not supply as much protein as animal sources.

Vegans can improve the protein content of their diet by including plenty of legumes such as soybeans and chickpeas, which have protein of almost as high quality as animal protein.

Combining foods from different groups also improves the quality of protein from nonanimal sources. For example, legumes complement grains; the combinations of beans with corn, beans with rice, and peanuts with wheat are all complete protein sources.

Avoiding Specific Deficiencies

Because the iron of animal protein is more absorbable than iron of plant origin, iron deficiency may develop in strict vegetarians unless food is selected carefully. Good plant sources of iron include legumes (especially soybeans), leafy green vegetables, whole-grain products, and dried fruits.

Vegetarians would do well to cook an occasional meal in a cast-iron pot, a good source of iron, which leaches from the pot into food.

A strict vegetarian diet is also likely to lead to calcium deficiency, because the milk group, a major source of calcium, is excluded. Good alternative sources of calcium are some dark-green, leafy vegetables, such as collards, kale, and dandelion, mustard, and turnip greens. Some calcium can also be obtained from broccoli, okra, rutabaga, legumes (especially soybeans), dried fruits, and some nuts (especially almonds).

In order for calcium to be absorbed properly, vitamin D is needed. Given enough exposure to sunlight, vitamin D is produced in the skin. If exposure is limited and the diet excludes such good animal sources of the vitamin a egg yolk, butter, liver, sardines, salmon, herring, and tuna, a vitamin D supplement may be needed.

The vitamin riboflavin is ordinarily well supplied by such sources as milk, meat, and eggs. Without these in the diet, a sufficient intake can be guaranteed by adding dried yeast to foods. Other good sources include cereals, whole-grain and enriched breads, legumes, broccoli, brussels sprouts, green leafy vegetables, okra, asparagus, and winter squash.

Vitamin B_{12} is the only nutrient very difficult to get from other than animal sources. It is essential for normal blood-cell formation and nerve functioning. Deficiencies can be avoided by the use of supplements containing the vitamin or with foods, such as breakfast cereals, which are fortified with vitamin B_{12}.

Fermented soybean products also can be a good source

of vitamin B_{12}. One such product, tempeh (an Indonesian bean cake sold in this country), is reported to be a particularly reliable source.

Is a Vegetarian Diet Healthier?

Many claims have been made that vegetarian diets are healthier, that vegetarians live longer and that vegetarianism protects against such degenerative diseases as cancer, high blood pressure, coronary heart disease, and diabetes. But there has been little evidence up to now to support the claims.

A vegetarian diet, however, may help with some health problems. For one thing, it is often lower in calories, and vegetarians have been found in some studies to weigh less for their height than nonvegetarians. Because of the amount of fiber in their diet, vegetarians are also less likely to have problems with constipation.

It is a fact, too, that a typical vegetarian diet is closer than the typical American nonvegetarian diet to some of the guidelines in the recent government publication, *Dietary Guidelines for Americans.* It is lower in saturated fats, higher in fiber, and has more complex carbohydrates.

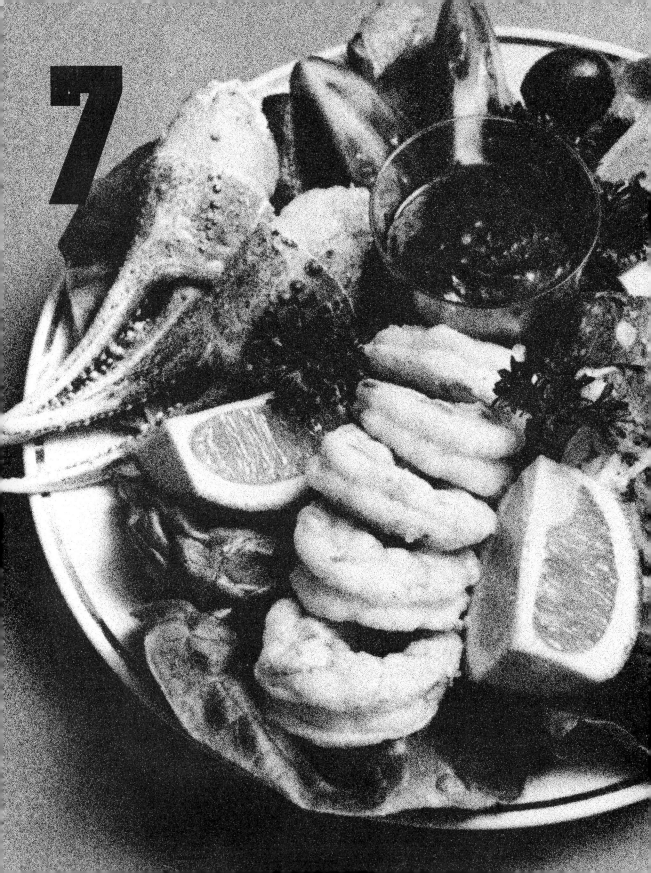

IDEAL DIET

Everything considered, what is the ideal diet? In general? For you in particular?

How do you achieve it at home?

How can you adhere to it in restaurants and when you travel?

What dividends can you reasonably expect from it?

Balance and Variety

It must be obvious that nutrition plays not only a vital role in health, but also a complex role. There is no one predominant nutrient or group of nutrients. There are dozens of them, including amino acids (in proteins), carbohydrates, fats, vitamins, and minerals. All are essential and interrelated. Let one be either deficient or present in excess, and others are affected. For example, without enough vitamin C in the diet, you may not absorb all the iron you need; with too much calcium in the diet, you may become zinc-deficient.

What we already know about nutrition may make it seem like a complex business—all the more so because of the complexity of its interrelationships—but we may not know a fraction of what there is to know about it. At any time,

All nutrients are interrelated. Let one be deficient or present in excess, and others are affected.

231

some basic new finding may be made—of a previously unknown vitamin or other essential nutrient, for example, or of a previously unsuspected interrelationship.

The more we know about nutritional complexities, the more one fact stands out: Except for certain specific problems—disease states for which special diets have been established as clearly helpful—the healthiest diet is balanced and varied.

Nature has a way of distributing largesse, and we are most likely to benefit by eating a variety of foods chosen from the major food groups.

If we do this—getting both balance and diversity rather than sameness—we are far less likely to suffer from deficiencies or excesses and almost certainly will enjoy the values of the still undiscovered.

Finding the Correct Balance

This is simply a matter of getting, in suitable servings each day, foods from each of the *basic four food groups* (see table on page 233). A balanced diet requires two servings each from the meat and meat substitutes group and the dairy products group and four servings each from the fruit and vegetables group and the grains group. By varying our choices within each group from day to day, we can have a healthy, balanced variety of foods, with neither too much nor too little of any valuable nutrient, either currently known or still to be identified.

H.K., a 36-year-old successful oil man, has found a way to add variety to his diet and ensure better health at the same time. He was concerned about his health because of cancer in his family; his father had died prematurely of colon cancer. Each year H.K. has a thorough physical examination at Executive Health Examiners. Last year he asked the physician to refer him to the nutritionist to discuss improvements in his diet.

He was proud that his present weight was only 15 pounds over his college weight, but he complained that his muscles were becoming "soft" and that a "spare tire" was developing around his middle. He loved to eat red meat,

THE BASIC FOUR FOOD GROUPS

The four groups	Nutrients supplied	Daily adult servings	One serving equals
Meat and meat substitutes: Beef, pork, lamb, veal, fish, poultry, eggs, organ meats, cheese, dry beans, lentils, peas, nuts	Protein, fat, iron, niacin, thiamine, vitamins B_{12} and E, copper, phosphorus	2	2 oz cooked lean meat, fish, or poultry; 2 eggs; 1 cup cooked dry beans, peas, or lentils; $\frac{1}{2}$ cup nuts or 4 tbsp peanut butter; 2 oz hard cheese; $\frac{1}{2}$ cup cottage cheese
Dairy products: Milk, yogurt, natural and processed cheeses, ice cream, ice milk, food products made with whole or skim milk	Protein, fat, calcium, riboflavin, vitamins A and D, zinc, magnesium	2	1 cup milk or yogurt; 1 oz cheese; $\frac{1}{2}$ cup cottage cheese, $\frac{1}{2}$ cup ice cream; 1 cup milk-based food (pudding, soup, or beverage)
Fruit and vegetables: All fruits and vegetables (fresh, frozen, canned, dried, and juices)	Carbohydrates, water, vitamins A and C, iron, magnesium	4	1 cup cut-up raw fruit or vegetable; 1 medium apple, banana, orange, tomato, or potato; $\frac{1}{2}$ melon or grapefruit; $\frac{1}{2}$ cup cooked vegetable or fruit; $\frac{1}{2}$ cup fruit or vegetable juice
Grains: Whole-grain or enriched flour, pasta, rice, cereal products	Carbohydrates, fat, protein, thiamine, niacin, vitamin E, calcium, iron, phosphorus, magnesium, zinc, copper	4	1 slice bread; 1 oz dry cereal; 1 roll or muffin; 1 pancake or waffle; $\frac{1}{2}$ cup rice, pasta, or cooked cereal

butter, eggs, cheese, and other high-fat foods plus sweet and salty snacks and desserts. He ate very little fiber, drank a lot of coffee and alcohol but only limited amounts of water, and complained of frequent constipation. There was little variety in his diet.

When the nutritionist showed H.K. results of epidemiologic studies linking cancer to elevated dietary fat, he became especially motivated to change his diet. After he incorporated more fiber into his daily diet and began drinking more water, his constipation disappeared. The nutritionist reminded him that fiber is worthless unless it is accompanied by enough fluid to increase its size and bulk.

Gradually H.K. ate fewer rich, fatty, and sweet foods and

selected more high-fiber foods, vegetables, and fruit, which gave much more variety to his diet than it had had before. He restricted his salty snacks, began exercising, and drank less alcohol. His muscles were strengthened, and his weight dropped slightly.

H.K. is doing everything he can to achieve his "ideal" diet. He feels good about his accomplishments and agrees with Executive Health Examiners that *prevention* is the best medication.

Going for Variety

If you are *not* in the habit of choosing the same few foods repeatedly from each food group—the same limited number of meats and fruits and vegetables, for example—you are doing well. If you *have* been restricting your diet in this manner, try to broaden your selection.

You may not like all foods, but you may find that you like some foods that you have never tried before and even some that you have tried but did not like in the past. Our taste buds change.

You may also find that some foods have a new interest for you when they are prepared in new ways (and there is no shortage of new ways to be found in the seemingly endless array of cookbooks that are available).

The greater the variety in your diet, the better it is for your health—and the greater the variety, you are likely to find, the greater your enjoyment as well.

What about . . . ?

Proteins Sure, they're important, but remember that only limited amounts are needed, that steaks and chops are not the only foods containing proteins, and that most Americans (97 percent according to some authorities) consume much more protein than is required, especially in the form of meat. It's fine for you to eat meat, but it would probably be prudent for you to decrease your intake of fat-rich meats and to increase your intake of fish, poultry, and lean meats.

If you eat 4 ounces of meat, you are getting 28 grams of protein—which is half of the U.S. recommended daily allowance (RDA) of protein for a 154-pound man. Add just a pint of milk, four slices of bread, half a cup of cereal, and a medium-sized potato, and you have the full 56-gram allowance.

Remember that protein, weight for weight, has the same number of calories as carbohydrates, but excess protein turns into fat and may contribute to obesity.

Fat and Cholesterol You need both; they play essential roles in the body. But there is almost no chance that you are not getting enough of them—just the reverse. With the American diet generally running to 42 percent fat, up from 32 percent earlier in the century, most of us would do well to decrease our fat intake by 25 percent.

Fat and cholesterol are interrelated. You will recall that not only do foods rich in cholesterol itself—egg yolks, shrimp, liver, kidney, and other organ meats, for example—raise blood cholesterol levels, so do saturated fats, which are found mainly in animal products, such as meat, butter, and cheese.

All the evidence indicates that it would be prudent for us to moderate our intake of cholesterol, to reduce our intake of saturated fats in favor of unsaturated fats (found in vegetable oils such as corn and safflower oil), and to moderate our total intake of fats, both saturated and unsaturated.

Carbohydrates Chances are you could consume more

of these undervalued essentials; most of us could. On an average, 46 percent of our calories come from carbohydrates, whereas once it was 60 percent. Our attention, however, should be directed to some, but not all, carbohydrates.

Currently, of the 46 percent of our energy that we receive from carbohydrates, 24 percent comes from sugar and only 22 percent comes from complex carbohydrates (starches). Very clearly, we need less sugar, and most of us could benefit from more of the complex carbohydrates found in fruits, vegetables, and cereal products, which also contain important vitamins, minerals, and dietary fiber.

Fiber Fiber can be found in the foods containing those valuable starches, the complex carbohydrates, that we just mentioned. If you eat enough of them, you don't have to add extra fiber to your diet.

Eating foods high in fiber tends to reduce symptoms of chronic constipation and diverticular disease and even symptoms of the most common of bowel complaints, irritable colon. It may also reduce the risk of developing cancer of the colon.

Sugar The average American consumption of almost 140 pounds of sugar a year has to be considered excessive. Beyond contributing significantly to dental decay, sugar contributes to obesity by providing us with a lot of empty calories without providing us with any vitamins or minerals. In short, sugar supplies us with nothing more than otherwise obtainable energy.

Insofar as obesity is a risk factor for atherosclerosis, coronary heart disease, and diabetes, excess sugar may also play a role in these diseases.

It would be prudent for us to use less of all sugars, including white, brown, and raw sugar and honey and syrups; to eat less of sugar-containing foods such as candy, soft drinks, ice cream, cakes, and cookies; to select fresh fruits or fruits canned without sugar or with light rather than heavy syrup; and to read food labels and recognize that if sucrose, glucose, maltose, dextrose, lactose, fructose, or corn syrup appear toward the top of the ingredient list, the product contains a large amount of sugar. And don't forget that sugar is one of the principal ingredients of alcohol.

Salt Moderate your use of it. Salt is a major hazard for anyone with high blood pressure or who is susceptible to salt's influence in promoting elevated blood pressure. There is no effective way yet of telling who is and who is not susceptible to this influence.

Some 17 percent of American adults have elevated blood pressure which, if uncontrolled, can be a major killer by contributing significantly to coronary heart disease, heart attacks, strokes, and kidney failure.

Keeping Your Weight in Line

A well-balanced and varied diet lends itself to maintaining desirable weight. It can—and should—be coupled with physical activity to maintain fitness.

There is no need for a daily weigh-in, but weighing once weekly is advisable. If you gain a pound or two in the course of a week, and especially if a further gain occurs the next week, it is best to take action.

You may need, very literally, to take action by increasing your physical activity, or you may need to cut down a bit on caloric intake, or both.

With 3, 4, or 5 pounds to take off, only a minimal dietary adjustment is needed. It could be simply a matter of a few cutbacks for several weeks or a month or two—one less of several daily pats of margarine and slices of bread, a slice less of bacon, or any of the other cutbacks noted in Table 3-6 that may be applicable.

If You Are Overweight Now

Say you are 10, 15, 30, or even more pounds over your desirable weight. Forego quick-loss diets and pay no attention to the latest wonder "high-this" or "low-that" diet.

You want to take off your excess weight while maintaining your health and to develop an eating pattern you can live with enjoyably for the rest of your life—not just take pounds off and gain them all back again.

This requires a balanced and varied diet, the kind we've been talking about here, so that you will achieve weight loss comfortably and be able to maintain that loss permanently.

A CONCISE REFERENCE GUIDE TO PRUDENT EATING

	Amt	Cal	Restricted	OK	Chol
Dairy Products					
Cheese:					
Cheddar, grated	1 tbsp	30	X		8
Cheddar, processed, 1 slice	1 oz	105	X		32
Cottage	1 oz	30		*	1
Cream	1 tbsp	55	X		9
Swiss Camembert	1 oz	105	X		41
Chocolate milk	8 oz	190	X		
Cocoa:					
Whole milk	8 oz	230	X		26
Skim milk	8 oz	150		*	
Cornstarch pudding	½ cup	138	X		17
Cream:					
Half-and-half (12% fat)	1 tbsp	20	X		6
Light; also sour cream (20% fat)	1 tbsp	35	X		10
Heavy (35% fat)	1 tbsp	55	X		18
Custard, baked or tapioca	½ cup	143	X		152
Egg:					
White	1	15		*	0
Whole	1 lg	80	X		234
Yolk	1	60	X		234
Ice cream, plain	½ cup	145	X		35
Ice milk	½ cup	143		†	6
Milk:					
Whole	8 oz	160	X		27
Skim (reconstituted or fortified)	8 oz	80		*	
Evaporated	1 tbsp	22	X		9
Pream	1 tsp	11	X		
Whipped topping (can)	1 tbsp	18	X		
Yogurt (partially skimmed milk)	8 oz	120		*	14
Fish and Seafood					
Clams, raw	3½ oz	49		†	150
Crab meat, canned or cooked	3½ oz	98		†	150
Fish sticks, breaded	1 piece	40		†	14
Herring	1 piece (25 g)	53	X		23
Ocean perch, breaded, deep fat fried	3½ oz	230		†	66
Oysters, raw (2 or 3 med)	1 oz	14		†	32
Salmon, pink, canned	3 oz	120	X		54
Salmon, red, smoked	3 oz	150	X		51
Sardines (drained)	1 oz	60	X		23
Shrimps	3½ oz	120		†	150
Tuna	3 oz	170	X		51
Fish: cooked, smoked, lean	3½ oz	130	X		70
Mixed Dishes, Soups, and Salads					
Baked beans:					
Canned, with pork	½ cup	165		†	4
With salt pork, homemade	½ cup	130	X		18
With oil, homemade	½ cup	195		X	
Borscht with sour cream	½ cup	50	X		6
Cheese blintzes, baked	1 oz	56	X		37
Chicken chow mein, noodles separate	½ cup	132		X	28
Chicken livers, chopped	2 oz	115	X		112
Chili:					
With beans, canned	1 cup	335		†	100
No beans, canned	1 cup	510	X		144
Chop suey:					
Lean pork	½ cup	100		†	42
Ground beef	½ cup	175	X		54
Chow mein noodles	1 cup	220		X	
Corned beef hash, canned	3 oz	120	X		36
Denver sandwich: fried eggs, ham	1 sandwich	318	X		274
Dumpling	1 oz	89	X		2
Egg roll, deep fat fried	1 piece (1 oz)	83	X		16
Gefilte fish	1 oz	37		X	19
Gravy:					
With beef fat and flour	1 tbsp	34	X		4
With oil and flour	1 tbsp	34		X	
Kreplach:					
Meat, boiled	1 oz	73	X		44
Cheese, boiled	1 oz	53	X		26
Macaroni and cheese	1 cup	485	X		88
Meat loaf	3 oz	305	X		135
Noodles and cottage cheese	½ cup	150		†	60
Potato:					
Pancakes	1 sm (2 oz)	68	X		24
Patty or cake	2 oz	106	X		56
Pot pie, 8 oz:					
Beef	½ pie	230	X		54
Poultry	½ pie	243		†	35
Pizza with tomato and cheese	3-in wedge	90	X		2
Rice:					
Pilaf	1 cup	235		†	28
Fried	½ cup	265	X		94
Salad:					
Chicken	3 oz	195		X	36
Kidney bean	½ cup	175		X	10
Potato, German	½ cup	125		†	6
Potato, with mayonnaise	½ cup	250		X	14
Shrimp	3 oz	95		†	80
Tuna or salmon (restaurant)	3 oz	145		X	36
Waldorf	½ cup	120		X	7
Salmon loaf	3 oz	148		†	108
Soup:					
Bean	1 cup	190		†	12

	Amt	Cal	Restricted	OK	Chol		Amt	Cal	Restricted	OK	Chol
Beef with meat	1 cup	100		†	4	French-fried in cottonseed oil					
Broth: bouillon, consommé, onion	1 cup	15		*		(5 pieces)	1 oz	78		X	
Clam chowder, no milk	1 cup	80		X	52	French-fried in hydrogenated fat					
Cream, canned (all varieties)	1 cup	200	X		40	(5 pieces)	1 oz	78	X		
Cream, homemade	1 cup	265	X		56	French-fried in corn oil					
Noodle or rice	1 cup	115		*	4	(5 pieces)	1 oz	78		X	
Pea	1 cup	140		*	36	French-fried, frozen					
Vegetable, tomato	1 cup	90		*		(5 pieces)	1 oz	78	X		
Spaghetti:						Mashed with milk and butter	½ cup	58	X		
With meat sauce	1 cup	285		†	28	Roasted	½ medium	82	X		
With tomato and cheese	1 cup	215		†	156	Scalloped	½ cup	120	X		
Stew:						Potato chips	5 lg	55	X		
Beef, vegetables	1 cup	185	X		108	Pumpkin, canned	½ cup	38		*	
Oyster, made with whole milk and butter	1 cup	200	X		256	Spinach	½ cup	23		*	
Tomato aspic	1 cup	70		*		Soybean sprouts, raw	½ cup	25		*	
Veal:						Squash:					
Curried	½ cup	200		†	96	Summer, diced	½ cup	18		*	
Scallopini (restaurant)	½ cup	320	X		106	Winter, baked or mashed	½ cup	48		*	
						Sweet potatoes:					
Vegetables						Boiled	½ medium	85		*	
Asparagus:						Candied	½ medium	148		†	
Fresh	½ cup	18		*		Tomatoes:					
Canned	½ cup	20		*		Raw	½ medium	15		*	
Beans:						Canned	½ cup	23		*	
Lima (small)	½ cup	75		*		Tomato catsup	1 tbsp	15		*	
Green or wax	½ cup	13		*		Turnips, diced	½ cup	20		*	
Beets, diced	½ cup	35		*							
Broccoli spears	½ cup	23		*		**Fruit**					
Brussels sprouts	½ cup	30		*		Fruit fresh, average	½ cup	58		*	
Cabbage:						Apple:					
Raw, shredded	½ cup	13		*		Fresh	1 medium	70		*	
Sauerkraut or plain cooked	½ cup	20		*		Juice	½ cup	63		*	
Coleslaw with dressing	¼ cup	35		*		Applesauce (also ½ pear), canned	¼ cup	45			
Carrots:						Apricots:					
Raw (½ med)	1 oz	10		*		Fresh	3	55		*	
Diced	½ cup	23		*		Canned (4 with 2 tbsp syrup)	4 halves	105		*	
Cauliflower	½ cup	15		*		Dried (¼ cup)	10 halves	98		†	
Corn:						Juice	½ cup	70		*	
Ear	1	65		*		Avocado	¼ cup	65			
Canned (all varieties)	½ cup	85		*		Banana	1 medium	85		*	
Greens, all except spinach	½ cup	84		*		Blueberries	½ cup	43		*	
Lettuce, celery, other salad vegetables	½ cup	6		*		Cantaloupe	¼ medium	20		*	
Okra	½ cup	30		*		Cherries, raw (8–10 lg)	½ cup	33		*	
Onions	½ cup	40		*		Cranberry sauce	1 tbsp	34		*	
Parsnips	½ cup	48		*		Dates: fresh, dried (3–4)	1 oz	80		*	
Peas:						Figs: fresh, dried	1 lg	60		*	
Green, fresh or frozen	½ cup	55		*		Fruit cocktail, heavy syrup	½ cup	98		*	
Green, canned	½ cup	85		*		Grapefruit:					
Potatoes:						Fresh	½ medium	50		*	
Boiled or baked	½ medium	45		*							

A CONCISE REFERENCE GUIDE TO PRUDENT EATING (Continued)

	Amt	Cal	Restricted	OK	Chol
Sections, raw	½ cup	38		*	
Juice, fresh	½ cup	48		*	
Juice, canned, sweetened	½ cup	65		*	
Grapes:					
15 malaga, 40 green seedless	½ cup	50		*	
Juice	½ cup	63		*	
Honeydew melon	½ cup	38		*	
Lemon juice	1 tbsp	5		*	
Lemonade, sweetened	½ cup	56		*	
Orange:					
Fresh	1 medium	70		*	
Juice: fresh, canned, or frozen	½ cup	56		*	
Peach:					
Fresh	1 medium	35		*	
Canned with juice	1 half	45		*	
Dried (4 med halves)	1 oz	75		*	
Juice	½ cup	70		*	
Pear, fresh	1 lg	100		*	
Pineapple:					
Fresh	½ cup	38		*	
Canned, sliced	1 slice	95		*	
Juice	½ cup	63		*	
Plum, fresh	1 lg	30		*	
Prunes, dried	4 medium	70		*	
Raisins	¼ cup	115		*	
Strawberries:					
Fresh	½ cup	28		*	
Frozen	¼ cup	60		*	
Watermelon, 4 by 4 in	1 piece	60		*	
Cereals, Breads, and Baked Goods				*	
Biscuits, baking powder	1 medium	130			2
Bread crumbs, dry, grated	1 tbsp	23		X	
Bread:					
Boston brown	1 slice	100		*	1
White, enriched	1 slice	60			1
White, unenriched;				*	
French; raisin	1 slice	60		*	1
Whole wheat	1 slice	55			1
Brownie, 2 by 2 in	1	124	X		39
Cake, without frosting:				*	
Angel food, 2-in wedge	1 piece	110		†	
Chiffon, 1¼-in wedge	1 piece	141			39
Cheese, 2 by 3 in	1 piece	196	X		51
Chocolate, plain, 2-in wedge	1 piece	144	X		39
Cereals:				*	
Dry, unsweetened	1 cup	110		*	
Dry, sweetened	1 cup	120			
Cookies, ½ in:					
medium fat	1	35		†	7
High fat	1	35		†	3
Chocolate chip	1	31		†	4
Peanut butter	1	32		†	3
Corn grits:					
Enriched	½ cup	60		*	
Unenriched	½ cup	60		*	
Corn meal, enriched	2 tbsp	66		*	
Corn muffins, cornbread	1 medium	155	X		32
Cracker:					
Graham	1 medium	28		*	
Saltine	1	18		*	
Ritz	1	11	X		1
Doughnut	1	135	X		27
Farina, enriched	½ cup	53		*	
Fig bar	1	55		†	
Flour, enriched	1 tbsp	25		*	
French toast with butter	1 slice	153	X		144
Matzo	1	56		†	1
Muffin:					
Plain	1	135	X		23
English	1 half	56		*	1
Oatmeal	1 cup	130		*	
Pancake:					
with hydrogenated fat	1 medium	60	X		23
with oil	1 medium	62		X	
Pasta: macaroni, noodles, spaghetti	1 cup	190		*	
Pie crust with shortening	⅐ crust	94	X		
Pie:					
Custard	1 piece	265	X		87
All fruit	1 piece	330	X		11
Lemon meringue	1 piece	300	X		59
Mince	1 piece	340	X		3
Pumpkin	1 piece	265	X		87
Popcorn, no fat added	½ cup	28		*	
Pretzels, sticks	5 sm	20		*	
Rice, instant	1 cup (cooked)	180		*	
Roll, hard	1 lg	160		*	2
Rye wafers, RyKrisp	2 pieces	43		*	
Strudel, all types	1 sm	165	X		6
Stuffing, bread:					
With hydrogenated fat	¼ cup	64	X		
With oil	¼ cup	68		X	
No added fat	¼ cup	36		*	
Waffle	1 medium	240	X		128
Beverages and Spirits					
Beer	8 oz	114		*	
Carbonated beverages, average	8 oz	105		*	

A CONCISE REFERENCE GUIDE
TO PRUDENT EATING (Continued)

	Amt	Cal	Restricted	OK	Chol
Cocktails:					
Grasshopper	4 oz	400			24
Manhattan	4 oz	270		*	
Martini	4 oz	310		*	
Old-fashioned	4 oz	345		*	
Whiskey sour	4 oz	285		*	
Ginger ale	8 oz	80		*	
Liqueur or fruit cordial	1 oz	95		*	
Rum	1 oz	95		*	
Wine:					
Light dry (12% to 14% alcohol)	4 oz	110		*	
Dry (20% alcohol)	4 oz	160		*	
Sweet (20% alcohol)	4 oz	180		*	
Candies, Sweets, Relishes, and Sauces					
Baking chocolate:		73	X		
Bitter	½ oz	68	X		
Sweet	½ oz				
Candy bar, average,		145	X		
chocolate covered	1 oz	60		†	7
Caramels	½ oz				
Cocoa powder,		7		*	
unsweetened	1 tsp				
Chocolate:		245	X		148
Soufflé	½ cup	145	X		
Milk (candy)	1 oz	60		*	
Syrup	1 tbsp	10		*	
Cornstarch	1 tsp				
Frosting:		50		*	
Cooked, ½ oz	1 tbsp	90	X		7
Chocolate	1 tbsp	90	X		8
Cream	1 tbsp	115	X		2
Fudge, plain	1 oz				
Gelatin:		35		*	
Powder	1 tbsp	78		*	
Dessert, plain	½ cup	86		*	
Dessert, with fruit	½ cup	110		*	
Hard candy, nonfat	1 oz				
Macaroon	1 sm	47	X		6
Olives:					
Green	3 lg	16		*	
Black	3 lg	21		*	
Parfait, chocolate	½ cup	216	X		96
Pickles:					
Dill	1 oz	4		*	
Sweet	1	20		*	
Postum, instant	2 tbsp	36		*	
Sauces:					
Barbecue with butter	1 tbsp	58	X	*	20
Chili or mustard	1 tbsp	15		*	
Chocolate, rich	1 tsp	46	X		3
Hollandaise with butter	1 tbsp	68	X		90
Meat (restaurant)	2 tbsp	41	X		9

	Amt	Cal	Restricted	OK	Chol
Tomato with oil, no meat	1 tbsp	19		X	
White with butter	1 tbsp	27	X		7
Sherbet	½ cup	118		*	4
Sugar:					
White, brown	1 tsp	17		*	
Confectioners	1 tbsp	31		*	
Spreads, Oils, and Fats					
Butter	1 tsp	17	X		7
Chicken fat	1 tsp	23		†	
Lard, bacon fat	1 tsp	23	X		3
Margarine:					
Average	1 tsp	17	X		
Modified	1 tsp	17		X	
Mayonnaise	1 tbsp	108		X	
Oils:					
Coconut, palm	1 tbsp	124	X		
Corn	1 tbsp	124		X	
Cottonseed	1 tbsp	124		X	
Olive	1 tbsp	124		†	
Peanut	1 tbsp	124		X	
Safflower	1 tbsp	124		X	
Soybean	1 tbsp	124		X	
Salad dressing:					
Cheese	1 tbsp	80		†	4
French	1 tbsp	60		X	
Mayonnaise-type	1 tbsp	65		X	8
Thousand Island	1 tbsp	90		X	12
Vegetable fat, hydrogenated	1 tbsp	124	X		
Nuts and Legumes					
Almonds, shelled (3–4)	⅛ oz	21		†	
Beans (navy, etc.):					
dried, canned	½ cup	115		X	
Brazil nuts (1)	⅛ oz	23		†	
Cashews, roasted (2)	⅛ oz	20	X		
Coconut, shredded	1 tbsp	25	X		
Cowpeas (black-eyed peas), cooked	½ cup	95		†	
Peanuts, roasted (4)	⅛ cup	21		X	
Peanut butter	1 tbsp	95		X	
Peas, split, cooked	½ cup	145		X	
Pecans, halves (3)	⅛ oz	24		X	
Pecans, chopped	1 tbsp (¼ oz)	50		X	
Walnuts, shelled, halves (2)	⅛ oz	23		X	
Meats and Poultry‡					
Beef:					
Barbecue	4 oz	380	X		144
Chipped or dried	2 oz	115		†	12

	Amt	Cal	Restricted	OK	Chol		Amt	Cal	Restricted	OK	Chol
Corned	4 oz	460	X		144	Chops, rib, lean only	4 oz	300		†	144
Corned, canned	2 oz	120	X		72	Ham, boiled	2 oz	170	X		72
Hamburger	4 oz	380	X		144	Ham, lean only	4 oz	380		†	144
Roast, sirloin tip,						Roast, lean	4 oz	380		†	144
lean only	4 oz	260		†	144	Salt	½ oz	102	X		26
Roast, pot	4 oz	380	X		144	Sausage	4 oz	460	X		144
Roast, rump, lean only	4 oz	260		†	144	Spareribs, 2 avg ribs	1 oz	144	X		36
Short ribs	4 oz	460	X		144	Steak, tenderloin	4 oz	300		†	144
Steak, flank	4 oz	260		†	144	Poultry:					
Steak, porterhouse	4 oz	460	X		144	With skin	3 oz	185		†	69
Steak, round	4 oz	260		†	144	No skin	3 oz	100		X	66
Steak, sirloin, lean only	4 oz	260		†	144	Chicken, canned	2 oz	115		X	46
Stew meat	4 oz	460	X		144	Duck, goose, etc.	4 oz	370	X		80
Very lean	4 oz	260		†	144	Veal	4 oz	260		†	144
Lamb:						Miscellaneous:					
Chop, loin, lean only	4 oz	260		†	144	Bologna, salami	1 oz	86	X		28
Leg of, lean only	4 oz	260		†	144	Frankfurter	1 avg	156	X		56
Stew meat	4 oz	460	X		144	Liver, fried in					
Very lean	4 oz	260		†	144	hydrogenated fat	3 oz	180	X		288
Pork:						Luncheon meats	1 oz	83	X		28
Bacon, regular sliced	1 slice	48	X		8	Organ meats	1 oz	41	X		96
Bacon, Canadian	4 oz	260		†	144	Salami, kosher	1 oz	103	X		36

* Little or no fat (but watch calories).
† Contains a moderate amount of cholesterol and saturated fat, or a relatively high number of calories. Moderate servings okay.
‡ Many of the beef, lamb, and pork cuts in the restricted category are okay if all visible fat is trimmed off and they are prepared by low-fat cooking methods.
Note: Chol = milligrams of cholesterol; X (under restricted) = restrict use (too much saturated fat); X (under OK) = high in polyunsaturated fat.
SOURCE: Adapted from *Project Health: Fat of the Land*, Medcom, New York, 1972.

The preceding quick-reference guide has been found valuable by many clients of Executive Health Examiners. It was prepared with the cooperation of Jeremiah Stamler, M.D., of Northwestern University Medical School. You can use it for quick checks not only on calories, but also on cholesterol and saturated fat in order to determine which foods are best restricted, which are approved, and those for which moderate servings are advisable.

Travel and Restaurant Dining

Dining out can present problems for weight control and for prudent, healthy nutrition, but the problems are far from insoluble. The principles that follow are those we advise for clients at Executive Health Examiners. They include those which many executives themselves have recommended on the basis of effective use.

Your Rights Dining in good restaurants, you have the right to be assertive, to ask questions about menu items— what is in them and how they are prepared—and to request reasonable substitutions. If good restaurants once looked askance at these queries, more and more no longer do in this era of increasing nutritional awareness. Also, special meals are available on airplanes if you order them in advance.

Drinks It makes good sense nutritionally—and as a way to maintain mental acuity—to replace martinis and similar drinks during business meals with mineral water, club soda, or even a wine spritzer, which contains only an ounce or two of wine and calorie-free soda water.

Premeal Nibbling Between the time you order and the time your food is served, you can consume a lot of calories and fats in breads and spreads. Instead of eating them, ask for a salad and ask that the dressing be served on the side. Eschew cream and cheese dressings in favor of vinegar and oil.

If you are having soup, make it a clear soup.

The Main Course and After Choose chicken, veal, and fish dishes rather than beef all the time. Avoid gravies and sauces or have them served on the side so that you can regulate how much of them you eat on your food.

Trim the fat from all meats, including poultry fat, which you get rid of by removing and discarding the skin.

You have the right to be assertive, to ask questions about menu items . . . and to request reasonable substitutions.

Don't add salt to food automatically; taste it first. Refrain from adding salt whenever possible.

Don't use butter—and ask for your baked potato without butter or sour cream.

Have vegetables whenever possible—but not fried or seasoned with butter, cooked in egg-yolk batter, or served with cheese or cream sauce.

Drink skim rather than whole milk, and use it in your coffee as a substitute for cream.

Choose fruit rather than baked goods for dessert.

Recognize that restaurant portions often are oversized, and don't finish a serving when it is too large.

Look for variety.

Shopping for Food

In the Meat Department Choose more fish and poultry. Both are as rich in protein as red meat, but they have less total fat and some polyunsaturated fat. If possible, eat fish at least twice a week. With whole wheat bread and tea or coffee, smoked fish—salmon, whitefish, haddock, cod, or herring—can make a nutritious and enjoyable breakfast, but eat it no more than once a week in order to keep your salt intake low. For dinner, grilled steaks of salmon, swordfish, or other fish, or baked whole fish, can provide nourishing protein with relatively little saturated fat and only a moderate amount of calories.

Choose veal before other meats. It is beef, but it has much less fat than other beef products. In buying beef, lamb, or pork, choose the leanest cuts possible (leg of lamb; less-marbled cuts of beef, which are often cheaper than other cuts).

Keep to a minimum the purchase of such fatty meats as sausage, bacon, pastrami, corned beef, and many cold cuts. Buy instead cold sliced chicken or turkey.

In the Dairy Department Switch to skim or low-fat milk in place of whole milk. They contain the same amount of calcium, protein, and vitamins as whole milk, but much less butterfat (usually 3.5 percent, or none at all). Both can be used in coffee, although you can also use evaporated skim milk or a dried skim-milk powder. You should know that many of the preparations sold as coffee lighteners are made from one vegetable oil, coconut oil, which is a saturated fat.

Switch from cheeses made with cream or whole milk to skim-milk cheeses. Also, avoid butter and shortenings in foods; choose foods—and recipes, if you cook yourself—that substitute polyunsaturated margarine and vegetable oils. (Polyunsaturated margarine can be substituted for butter in *any* recipe.) An acceptable margarine would be one that lists liquid corn oil as its first ingredient.

Breads and Cereals Buy whole wheat or other whole-grain breads—which are rich in fiber—rather than white bread. Avoid butter rolls and commercial cakes, doughnuts, and muffins, which are usually baked with saturated fats. It is preferable that homemade bread, pastries, cakes, and biscuits be made with whole wheat, rather than white, flour. Choose unsugared cereals, preferably, those high in fiber, many of which are labeled as including "bran" or "oats."

Fruits and Vegetables Keep some fresh fruit and cleaned vegetables ready to eat as low-calorie snacks. Buy fresh fruit for dessert, to be eaten by itself or as a topping on frozen yogurt or sugarless gelatin.

Promoting Good Nutrition at Home

A Word to Spouses

Like many if not most executives—and, indeed, most Americans—the executive in your family may need to do one or more of a number of things to improve his or her diet. The objectives that both of you should have in mind are bringing or keeping weight under control, improving general health, and reducing the risk of heart disease and other serious diseases.

Your spouse may need—at home, on business lunches, and on other dining-out occasions—to eat better-balanced and more varied meals, to eat smaller portions, and to reduce the intake of such things as cholesterol, saturated fat, total fat, salt, and highly refined foods, all of which can be undesirable in excess.

You can—and undoubtedly will want to—help with all of this. Bear in mind that the kind of eating which is sensible for your husband or wife—and which can be made pleasant as well—can be sensible, healthy, and pleasant for you and the rest of your family.

Certainly, all the suggestions that follow will not be new to you, but given the increased interest of your husband or wife in good and prudent nutrition, you may find it easier to put them into practice.

A Word to Executives

Do not expect your spouse to keep this diet for you. It is your responsibility, and you are more likely to stay with it if you accept that fact from the start.

If your spouse works too, or is also an executive, he or she may also need assistance in staying on a diet, though the same self-responsibility applies to him or her as applies to you. However, dieting is always easier when it's a family affair.

Food Preparation

Vegetables and Fruits Handle them as little as possible and don't prepare them far ahead of time. Wash them quickly; don't soak them. Don't overdo peeling, because there are nutrients and fiber in the skin too; cook them whole, with skins on, whenever possible. Peeling and slicing can cause as much as a 50 percent loss of vitamin C.

Avoid thawing frozen vegetables and fruits until immediately before you are ready to cook or eat them; they can lose much of their nutrients otherwise.

Don't drain the liquid from canned vegetables. It contains as much as 40 percent of the vitamin C and one-third of the thiamine and riboflavin. Cook with it and save what is left for soups and sauces.

Avoid trimming such leafy vegetables as lettuce and cabbage; nutrient concentration tends to be greatest in the outer leaves.

Don't overcook frozen or canned vegetables; they have already been parboiled.

In cooking a fresh vegetable or fruit, drop it into already boiling water. (At high temperatures, because of the effect of an enzyme system in the foods, there is less destruction of vitamin C.) Cover the pot, bring the water to a boil again, and cook until tender but still firm. Better yet, cook vegetables and fruit in a steamer, because they retain even more of their vitamins when they're steamed than when they're boiled.

Don't use baking soda in cooking yellow or green vegetables; it destroys vitamins.

Don't leave vegetables in water or over heat once they are cooked. The cooking should be timed so that they can be served as soon as they are done. Continued heating speeds the destruction of vitamins.

Serve leftover vegetables such as asparagus, beets, peas, and beans in a salad the next day instead of reheating them, which causes more loss of nutrients.

Keep fruit at room temperature until ripe; then refrigerate it to conserve nutrients.

Orange juice is good for you, but remember that a whole orange provides more vitamins and fiber than juice; even the core and peel are high in valuable nutrients.

Meats The higher the cooking temperature, the greater the shrinking and drying—and also the loss of nutrients. Cook meat at moderate temperatures, 300 to 350°F, and don't overcook it. That also applies to pork, which, because of the possibility of trichinosis, many people "cook to death." Trichinae are destroyed at 140°F, so pork cooked at 325°F for 30 minutes a pound is safe—and more nutritious.

Roasting and broiling are the best ways of cooking meat from the standpoint of nutrient retention. During broiling, moreover, much of the fat drips off and can be discarded. Frying may actually double the calorie count.

When roasting, it is advisable to use a rack so the meat does not sit in the drippings while cooking. Low-temperature (325 to 350°F) roasting is best for flavor and also allows more fat to come out of the meat; higher temperatures tend to seal the fat in. Instead of basting with drippings (which contain fat) during roasting, try using wine, fruit juice, or broth to keep the meat moist and add an interesting flavor besides.

Roast turkey or chicken with a few onions, carrots, or

other vegetables in the cavity to add flavor, and bake stuffings separately, using fat-free broth to flavor them. Stuffing in poultry absorbs a lot of fat.

Fish Broil or bake fish at 400°F, leaving the skin on to prevent loss of juices and nutrients.

Poaching can produce a mild-flavored fish with the smallest amount of fat. For the poaching liquid, use a small amount of water, white wine, and some onions and herbs. Simmer the fish; don't let the poaching liquid boil or it may cause the fish to break up.

Cook fish only until it flakes easily; further cooking will make it dry and tough.

Steam lobsters and crabs in their shells to preserve nutrients. Shrimp can be shelled with little nutrient loss, since their cooking time is only 3 to 5 minutes.

Menu Planning

Try for a balanced diet with the appropriate number of daily servings from each of the four basic food groups. Even if it is difficult to persuade yourself to eat more grains, fruits, and vegetables, the results will make the effort worthwhile. If they are served in new ways, that may increase their appeal. If you can, get your family members to eat more raw fruit and vegetables, too.

Try for variety. As we noted earlier in this book, variety is the only practical way to ensure adequate intake of all known—and still unknown—nutrients while avoiding excesses of any one of them.

Also, try to gradually increase the use of herbs and spices in your food, including garlic and freshly ground pepper, as a way to enhance food flavors and minimize the use of salt. Even if you do not use more herbs and spices, try to cut down as much as possible the use of salt in the preparation of your food and at the table.

Eggs in moderation are good food. Moderation means at most four per person per week, and, according to some authorities better two than four—egg yolks, that is. They contain the cholesterol. With recipes calling for eggs, cooks have

AN ALTERNATIVE AMERICAN DIET PLAN

Low in Fat, Low in Cholesterol, Low in Sugar

Meal		Day					
	1	2	3	4	5	6	7
Breakfast	Apple wedges Steel-cut oatmeal with skim milk Cracked wheat toast with farmer's cheese	Fresh fruit and yogurt shake Homemade bran muffin	¼ honeydew melon with cottage cheese Walnut carrot bread	Broiled grapefruit Breakfast pizza (low-fat ricotta on English muffins)	Fresh juice Bran flakes with skim milk Fruit and nut cottage cheese sandwich	Cantaloupe with blueberries Tofu spread on cinnamon raisin English muffin	Orange slices Wheat germ pancakes
Lunch	Gazpacho soup Turkey sandwich on rye bread	Tomato stuffed with curried crabmeat	Chinese vegetables and tofu over rice Mango slices	Linguini with red clam sauce Tossed green salad	Peanut butter and alfalfa sprouts on corn molasses bread	Curried chicken salad with grapes	Tomato juice Bagels with farmer's cheese and smoked salmon
Dinner	Clam chowder* Salmon with dill sauce Green beans with water chestnuts Cold orange soufflé	Pasta with tomato sauce Veal scallopini marsala Broccoli Italian style Baked apple in cider	Guacamole with toasted (not fried) corn tortilla triangles Red snapper Crook neck squash with herbs Fruit-filled orange	Cream of asparagus soup* Sherry-roasted Cornish hen Fresh vegetable stuffing Raspberry sherbet	Melon wedge Osso bucco Milanese with whole wheat pasta Arrugula and endive salad Special pumpkin pie	Mushroom pâté Halibut teriyaki over brown rice Harvard beets Pineapple au kirsch	Vegetarian black bean soup Sesame Chicken Asparagus spears with pimento strips Bananas flambé with rum

* Made with skim milk.

HERBS AND SPICES

Herb or spice*	How it is available	How it tastes	How it is used
Allspice	Whole or ground	Like a blend of cinnamon, nutmeg and cloves	Spices meat, fish, seafood dishes, soups, juices, fruits, spicy sauces, spinach, turnips, peas, red and yellow vegetables
Anise	Whole or ground	Aromatic, sweet licorice flavor	Sweet rolls, breads, fruit pies, and fillings; sparingly in fruit stews, shellfish dishes, carrots, beets, cottage cheese
Basil, sweet	Fresh, whole or ground	Aromatic, mild mint-licorice flavor	Meat, fish, seafood dishes, eggs, soups, stews, sauces, salads, tomato dishes, most vegetables, fruit compotes
Bay	Dried whole leaves, ground	Aromatic, woodsy, pleasantly bitter	Meat, game, poultry, stews, fish, shellfish, chowders, soups, pickled meats and vegetables, gravies, marinades
Burnet	Fresh, dried leaves	Delicate cucumber flavor	Soups, salads, dressings, most vegetables, beverages, as a garnish
Caraway	Whole or ground, seed	Leaves and root delicately flavored, seeds sharp and pungent	Beans, beets, cabbage soup, breads, cookies, dips, a variety of meats, casseroles, dressings, cottage cheese, cheese spreads, sauerbraten
Cardamom	Whole or ground, seed	Mild, pleasant ginger flavor	Pastries, pies, cookies, jellies, fruit dishes, sweet potatoes, pumpkin
Cayenne	Ground	Blend of hottest chili peppers	Sparingly in sauces, meat or seafood dishes, casseroles, soups, curries, stews, Mexican recipes, vegetables, cottage and cream cheeses
Chervil	Fresh, whole	Delicate parsley flavor	Soups, salads, stews, meats, fish, garnishes, eggs, sauces, dressings, vegetables, cottage cheese
Chili powder	Powder	Blend of chilies and spices	Sparingly in Mexican dishes, meats, stews, soups, cocktail sauces, eggs, seafoods, relishes, dressings
Chives	Fresh, frozen, dried	Delicate onion flavor	As an ingredient or garnish for any dish complemented by this flavor
Cinnamon	Whole sticks or ground	Warm, spicy flavor	Pastries, desserts, puddings, fruits, spiced beverages, pork, chicken, stews, sweet potatoes, carrots, squash
Cloves	Whole or ground	Hot, spicy, penetrating	Sparingly with pork, in soups, desserts, fruits, sauces, baked beans, candied sweet potatoes, carrots, squash
Coriander	Whole or ground, seed	Pleasant lemon-orange flavor	Pastries, cookies, cream or pea soups, Spanish dishes, dressings, spiced dishes, salads, cheeses, meats
Cumin	Ground, seed	Warm, distinctive, salty-sweet, reminiscent of caraway	Meat loaf, chili, fish, soft cheeses, deviled eggs, stews, beans, cabbage, fruit pies, rice, Oriental meat cookery

HERBS AND SPICES
(Continued)

Herb or spice*	How it is available	How it tastes	How it is used
Curry	Powder	Combination of many spices, warm, fragrant, exotic, combinations vary	Meats, sauces, stews, soups, fruits, eggs, fish, shellfish, poultry, creamed and scalloped vegetables, dressings, cream or cottage cheeses
Dill	Fresh, whole or ground, seed	Aromatic, somewhat like caraway, but milder and sweeter	Seafood, meat, poultry, spreads, dips, dressings, cream or cottage cheeses, potato salads, many vegetables, soups, chowders
Fennel	Whole or ground, seed	Pleasant licorice flavor, somewhat like anise	Breads, rolls, sweet pastries, cookies, apples, stews, pork, squash, eggs, fish, beets, cabbage
Ginger	Fresh, whole root, ground, crystallized	Aromatic, sweet, spicy, penetrating	Cakes, pies, cookies, chutneys, curries, beverages, fruits, meats, poultry, stews, dressings, cheese dishes
Mace	Whole or ground	This dried pulp of nutmeg kernel has a strong nutmeg flavor	Chicken, creamed fish, fish sauces, cakes, cookies, spiced doughs, jellies, beverages, yellow vegetables, cheese dishes, desserts, toppings
Marjoram	Fresh, whole or ground	Faintly like sage, slight mint aftertaste, delicate	Pork, lamb, beef, game fish, fish sauces, poultry, chowders, soup, stews, sauces, cottage or cream cheeses, omelets, soufflés, green salads, many vegetables
Mint	Fresh, dried	Fruity, aromatic, distinctive flavor	Lamb, veal, fish, soup, fruit, desserts, cottage or cream cheeses, sauces, salads, cabbage, carrots, beans, potatoes
Mustard	Fresh, whole or ground	Sharp, hot, very pungent	Salads, dressings, eggs, sauces, fish, spreads, soups, many vegetables
Nutmeg	Whole or ground	Spicy, sweet, pleasant	Desserts of all kinds, stews, sauces, cream dishes, soups, fruits, beverages, ground meats, many vegetables
Oregano (wild marjoram)	Fresh, whole or ground	More pungent than marjoram, but similar, reminiscent of thyme	Italian cooking, Mexican cooking, spaghetti, tomato sauces, soups, meats, fish, poultry, eggs, omelets, spreads, dips, many vegetables, green salads, mushroom dishes
Parsley	Fresh, dried flakes	Sweet, mildly spicy, refreshing	As a garnish, in soups, spreads, dips, stews, butters, on all meats, poultry, fish, most vegetables, omelets, eggs, herb breads, salads
Poppy seed	Tiny whole dried seed	Nut flavor	Breads, rolls, cakes, soups, cookies, dressings, cottage or cream cheeses, noodles, many vegetables, fruits, deviled eggs, stuffings
Rosemary	Fresh, whole	Refreshing, piny, resinous, pungent	Sparingly in meats, game, poultry, soups, fruits, stuffings, eggs, omelets, herb breads, sauces, green salads, marinades, vegetables

HERBS AND SPICES
(Continued)

Herb or spice*	How it is available	How it tastes	How it is used
Saffron	Whole or ground	Exotic, delicate, pleasantly bittersweet	Expensive but a little goes far; use for color and flavor in rice dishes, potatoes, rolls, breads, fish, stew, veal, chicken, bouillabaisse, curries, scrambled eggs, cream cheese, cream soups, sauces
Sage	Fresh, whole or rubbed	Pungent, warm, astringent	Sparingly in pork dishes, fish, veal, lamb, stuffings, cheese dips, fish chowders, consommé, cream soups, gravies, green salads, tomatoes, carrots, lima beans, peas, onions, brussels sprouts, eggplant
Savory	Fresh, whole or ground	Warm, aromatic resinous, delicate sage flavor; winter savory stronger than summer savory	Egg dishes, salads, soups, seafoods, pork, lamb, veal, poultry, tomatoes, beans, beets, cabbage, peas, lentils, summer squash, artichokes, rice, barbecue dishes, stuffings
Sesame	Whole seed	Toasted, it has a nutlike flavor	Breads, rolls, cookies, fish, lamb, eggs, fruit or vegetable salads, chicken, thick soups, vegetables, casseroles, toppings, noodles, candies
Tarragon	Fresh, whole or ground	Licorice-anise flavor, pleasant, slightly bitter	Sparingly in egg dishes, fish, shellfish, veal, poultry, chowders, chicken, soups, butters, vinegar, sauces, marinades, beans, beets, cabbage, cauliflower, broccoli, vegetable juices, fresh sprigs in salads
Thyme	Fresh, whole or ground	Strong, pleasant, pungent clove flavor	Sparingly in fish, gumbo, shellfish, soups, meats, poultry, tomato juice or sauces, cheeses, eggs, sauces, fricasees, tomatoes, artichokes, beets, beans, mushrooms, potatoes, onions, carrots
Turmeric	Whole or ground	Aromatic, warm, mild	Substitutes for saffron in salads, salad dressings, butters, creamed eggs, fish, curries, rice dishes without saffron, vegetables, used partially for its orange color
Watercress	Fresh	Pleasing, peppery	Garnish or ingredient in salads, fruit or vegetable cocktails, soups, cottage cheese, spreads, egg dishes, or sprinkled on vegetables or sauces

* Approximately ⅓ tsp ground herbs or 1 tsp dried herbs is equal in strength to 1 tbsp fresh herbs.

> Variety is the only practical way to assure an adequate intake of all known—and still unknown—nutrients while avoiding excesses of any one of them.

been successfully using two egg whites, with a little oil, for each whole egg.

Plan for moderate rather than oversized portions. Servings should be smaller than many people realize. Note, for example, that just 2 ounces of cooked lean meat, fish, or poultry counts as a serving, which means that 4 ounces of meat in the course of a day is quite sufficient for an adult. One helpful way of achieving satisfaction with more moderate portions than customary is to encourage mealtime conversation as a way of slowing down eating. Eating slowly can lead to more enjoyment of food, and it gives the appetite a chance to be satiated before there is overeating.

It can also be helpful, if servings look small, to use smaller plates. Plates with rims and heavy patterns tend to make portions of food look more generous.

A Quick Course in Reading Food Labels

With few exceptions, food product labels include a list of ingredients. Many also carry a nutrition information panel.

> Encourage mealtime conversation as a way of slowing down eating—it can lead to more enjoyment of food.

The Ingredient List

This shows the ingredients in descending order of quantity in the recipe, main ingredient first. If the list for a frozen turkey dinner, for example, reads "potatoes, carrots, turkey," you are getting more vegetables than meat.

You can also figure that when sugar or some other sweetener is one of the first two or three ingredients of a product, there could be more sugar present than is nutritionally desirable. Note, too, that different kinds of sugars are listed separately, so you should look through the list for all such ingredients as honey, dextrose, corn syrup, corn sweetener, invert sugar, molasses, etc.

Ingredient lists give other useful information too. Here, for example, is a list for a chocolate chip cookie product:

> INGREDIENTS: Flour, chocolate, sugar, blend of partially hydrogenated vegetable shortening, (may contain partially hydrogenated soybean, cottonseed and/or palm oils), eggs, corn syrup, molasses, water, salt, sodium bicarbonate, natural and artificial flavors.

You can see that the major nutrients are carbohydrates (starches from flour, and sugars from corn syrup and molasses as well as common sugar) and fats (from chocolate, shortening, and eggs).

The flour is unenriched (without added B vitamins or iron), and the oils have been partially hydrogenated to improve their shortening properties, which means that the level of saturated fat has been somewhat increased and the level of polyunsaturated fat decreased.

Because of the salt and sodium bicarbonate content, such cookies—the recipe is a typical one for chocolate chip cookies—should be eaten very sparingly by anyone on a low-sodium diet and also by anyone on a cholesterol-fat-controlled diet, because of the chocolate, shortening, and eggs.

Particular attention should be paid to whether an ingredient list includes coconut or palm oil, both of which are more saturated than animal fats, or whether the list simply lists vegetable oil without indicating the kind, in which case it is likely to be coconut or palm oil.

The Nutrition Information Panel

This panel provides additional important data.

*   *Nutrition information is given for one-serving quantities, and the size of a serving (for example, 1 cup or 2 ounces or 2 tablespoons) is given along with the number of servings per container.*

    The number of calories per serving is listed, and the amount in grams (1 ounce = 28 grams) of protein, carbohydrates, and fats.

*   *Protein is listed both in grams and as a percentage of the U.S. recommended daily allowance (RDA) for protein.*

*   *The percentage of the RDA must also be listed for seven vitamins and minerals—vitamins A and C, thiamine, riboflavin, niacin, calcium, and iron.*

*   *Twelve other vitamins and minerals may also be listed—vitamins D, E, B_6, and B_{12}, folic acid (folacin), phosphorus, iodine, magnesium, zinc, copper, biotin, and pantothenic acid.*

*   *Optionally, the panel may also list the percentage of calories from fat and the amounts of fatty acids, cholesterol, and sodium.*

Here, for example, is the nutrition information panel from a jar of peanut butter:

NUTRITION INFORMATION PER SERVING

Serving size 2 tbsp (32 g)	Cholesterol* (0 mg/100 g)
	0 mg
Servings per container 10	Sodium (420 mg/100 g)
	150 mg
Calories 190	Percentage of U.S.
Protein 9 g	recommended daily
Carbohydrates 4 g	allowances (U.S. RDA)

* Information on fat and cholesterol content is provided for individuals who, on the advice of a physician, are modifying their total dietary intake of fat and/or cholesterol.

Fat 17 g
% of calories from
    fat* 74%
Polyunsaturated* 5 g
Saturated* 3 g

Protein 15% Niacin 20%
Iron 2%
Contains less than 2% of
    the U.S. RDA of vitamin A,
    vitamin C, thiamine,
    riboflavin, and calcium.

Using Nutrition Labels

The labels have a number of practical values. You can use them to:

* *Identify foods that are major sources for specific nutrients.*

* *Compare the nutrient composition of varied food items.*

* *Choose foods offering the best nutritional value for the money.*

* *Choose foods offering the best nutritional value considering the number of calories consumed.*

* *Assess the nutritional adequacy of one day's meals.*

* *Make substitutions or additions to improve your diet and choose food for a medically recommended special diet, such as one low in sodium.*

A Final Word

Nutrition is still a very young science, and there is much yet to be learned about it. What we are counseling encompasses

---

If what we are counseling had to be summed up in just one word, the word would be *moderation.*

---

what is known and leaves room for what is still to be discovered.

If what we are counseling had to be summed up in just one word, the word would be *moderation.* Until everything there is to be known about nutrition is, in fact, known—and quite possibly even then—moderation, with all that it means, is a fine practical guide to good nutrition.

Everything we know indicates that nutritional deficiencies, excesses, and imbalances play significant roles in many conditions, especially degenerative diseases. All the evidence points to the importance of sound nutrition in maintaining both mental and physical health.

Good nutrition, desirable for all, can be highly critical for executives who are under stress, lead extremely busy lives, need their wits about them at all times, and obviously need to maintain their health in order to advance in their careers.

Use our "Concise Reference Guide to Prudent Eating" for important information on the calorie and cholesterol contents of numerous foods.

If you are really well-nourished now, you probably already know the benefits—or, if you have only suspected them before, you should realize what they are now from what you've read here. If you have been less than well-nourished, we are confident that the information in this book will have been a revelation to you and will have shown you the direction to a healthier—and happier—life.

There can be no guarantees, of course, that you will live longer because of improved nutrition, although it is certainly a possibility. We are sure, however, that you will take well-justified pride—and pleasure—in feeling more fit and vigorous as the result of good nutrition.

WHEN SHOPPING FOR COMMERCIALLY PREPARED CAKES AND SNACKS, READ THE LABEL CAREFULLY

A case in point:

Ingredients: Sugar, enriched flour, eggs, corn syrup, dextrose, skim milk, whey, leavening, salt, starch, corn flour, mono- and diglycerides, sodium caseinate, polysorbate 60, artificial color and flavor, sorbic acid.

ACKNOWLEDGMENTS

Page 6, Myron Winick, M.D., "Nutrition in Clinical Practice," *Modern Medicine*, September 1977. Reprinted by permission of Modern Medicine Publishing Company and Myron Winick, M.D.

Page 14, by permission of Frederick J. Stare, M.D.

Page 16, A. H. Hayes, *The New York Times*, June 19, 1981 Copyright © by the New York Times Company. Reprinted by permission.

Page 17, R. S. Schweiker, *The New York Times*, June 12, 1981. Copyright © by the New York Times Company. Reprinted by permission.

Page 27, "Low-Fat Protein Foods Table," *Nutrition & Health*, 1(5):4, 1979. Reprinted by permission of the Institute of Human Nutrition.

Pages 36–38, 40, from *Nutrition* by Cheryl Corbin, M.S., R.D. Copyright © 1980 by Preventive Medicine Institute/Strang Clinic. Reprinted by permission of Holt, Rinehart and Winston, Publishers.

Pages 42–43, "Snack Food Chart," *Nutrition & Health*, 2(3):4–5, 1980. Reprinted by permission of the Institute of Human Nutrition.

Page 47, Robert E. Fuiz, M.D., *Project Health: The Fat of the Land*, Medcom, New York, 1972. Reprinted by permission of Medcom, Inc.

Page 48, by permission of RoseAnn Shorey, M.D.

Page 48, by permission of Mary B. McCann, M.D.

Page 48, Margaret Mackenzie, M.D., "Obesity as Failure in the American Culture," *Obesity & Bariatric Medicine*, Vol. 5, No. 4, 1976.

Page 55, George A. Bray, "Body Mass Index Nomogram," *International Journal of Obesity*, 2:1, 1978. Reprinted by permission of the *International Journal of Obesity* and George A. Bray.

Page 56, reproduced from "Recommended Dietary Allowances," (9th Edition) 1980, by permission of the National Academy of Sciences, Washington, D.C.

Page 74, G. A. Levey, *Vegetarian Times*, 6:28, 1980; adapted from Frank Konishi, "Food Energy Equivalents of Various Activities." Copyright © The American Dietetic Association. Reprinted by permission from *Journal of the American Dietetic Association*, Vol. 46:186, 1965.

Page 90, photos courtesy of United Airlines.

Page 109, "Salt Cycle Chart," *Nutrition & Health*, 1(3):3, 1979. Reprinted by permission of the Institute of Human Nutrition.

Page 110, "Salt Intake Chart," *Nutrition & Health*, 1(3):4, 1979; adapted from J. D. Krudsen and L. K. Dahl, *Postgraduate Medical Journal*, 42:148–152, 1966. Reprinted by permission of the Institute of Human Nutrition.

Pages 113, 114, 115, from *Nutrition* by Cheryl Corbin, M.S., R.D. Copyright © 1980 by Preventive Medicine Institute/Strang Clinic. Reprinted by permission of Holt, Rinehart and Winston, Publishers.

Page 116, Donald S. Silverberg, M.D., "Treating Hypertension with Diet," *Consultant*, July 1980. Reprinted by permission of Cliggott Publishing Company.

Pages 117–120, "Sodium Restriction Chart" (table and diet), *Nutrition & Health*, 1(3):4–5, 1979. Reprinted by permission of the Institute of Human Nutrition.

Page 129, chart on "The Effect of One Cigarette in Patients with Coronary Artery Disease," in O. Gillie and D. Mercer (eds.), *The Complete Book of Body Maintenance*. Reprinted by permission of W. W. Norton & Company, Inc.

Page 133, J. Stamler, "Population Studies," in R. I. Levy et al. (eds.), *Nutrition, Lipids and Coronary Heart Disease.* Copyright © 1979 by Raven Press, New York. Reprinted by permission of Raven Press.

Pages 152, 155, reproduced from "Recommended Dietary Allowances," (9th Edition) 1980, by permission of the National Academy of Sciences, Washington, D.C.

Page 160, Dr. Neville Colman, *Journal of the American Medical Association*, 243:2473, 1980. Copyright © 1980, American Medical Association. Reprinted by permission of the American Medical Association.

Page 166, "Calcium/Phosphorus Content and Ratio Chart," *Nutrition & Health*, 1(3):4, 1979. Reprinted by permission of the Institute of Human Nutrition.

Pages 180–181, excerpted by permission from *Consumer Reports*, July 1980. Copyright © by Consumers Union of United States, Inc., Mount Vernon, New York 10550.

Pages 181, 184, 186–187, Marilyn Stephenson, *FDA Consumer*, HEW Publication (FDA), July–August 1978.

Page 182, Myron Winick, M.D., *Medical World News*, August 22, 1977. Reprinted by permission of HEI Publishing, Inc.

Page 182, *FDA Consumer*, HEW Publication (FDA) 79-2108, July 1978.

Pages 185–186, Thomas H. Jukes, Ph.D. and Stephen Barrett, M.D., in *The Health Robbers*, Stephen Barrett, M.D. and Gilda Knight (eds.). Copyright © 1976 by George F. Stickley Company, Philadelphia. Reprinted by permission of George F. Stickley Company.

Page 187, Victor D. Herbert, M.D., *Nutrition Cultism: Facts & Fictions.* Copyright © 1981 by George F. Stickley Company, Philadelphia. Reprinted by permission of George F. Stickley Company.

Pages 187–188, "Where to Get Trustworthy Advice," *The New York Times*, March 25, 1981. Copyright © 1981 by The New York Times Company. Reprinted by permission.

Pages 189–190, Copyright © by Consumers Union of United States, Inc., Mount Vernon, New York 10550. Excerpted by permission from *Consumer Reports*, July 1980.

Page 196, Peter G. Lindner, M.D., "Guest Editorial," *Obesity & Bariatric Medicine*, Vol. 7, No. 4, 1978.

Page 201, "Fiber Diets," *Nutrition & Health*, 1(5):5–6, 1979. Reprinted by permission of the Institute of Human Nutrition.

Page 202, "Dietary Fiber Table," adapted from tables published in the Marabou Symposium, *Food and Fiber.*

Page 210, Tavia Gordon and Charles Kaelber, M.D., *Alcohol, Drug Abuse, and Mental Health Administration News*, Vol. 6, No. 20, October 1980. Reprinted by permission of *ADAMHA News.*

Page 210, "Capsule & Comment" (Gene Stollerman, M.D., ed.) *Hospital Practice*, January 1981. Reproduced with permission from HP Publishing, Inc.

Page 211, Arthur L. Klatsky, M.D., *Medical Tribune*, Vol. 21, No. 10, March 1980. Reprinted by permission of Medical Tribune, Inc.

Page 212, "Alcohol and Calories Chart," *A Maximal Approach to the Dietary Treatment of the Hyperlipidemias*, Subcommittee on Diet and Hyperlipidemia, Council on Arteriosclerosis, American Heart Association, 1973. Reprinted with permission of the American Heart Association.

Page 220, "Caffeine Content of Foods and Drugs Chart," *The Health Effects of Caffeine*, American Council of Science and Health, March 1981. Reprinted by permission of American Council of Science and Health.

INDEX

Coloring agents, 174–176, 190
  polymeric, 180
Common cold, effects of vitamin C on, 154–156
Complete protein source, defined, 24
Complex carbohydrates (see Carbohydrates)
Congestive heart failure, hypertension and, 104
Connolly, Cyril, 50
Constipation, 233
  dietary fiber and, 37, 196–197, 229, 236
  hypercalcemia and, 167
Consumer Reports (magazine), 189
Controlled-carbohydrate, modified-fat, moderately re-
  stricted cholesterol diet, 144
Convulsions due to mineral deficiencies, 168, 171
Cooking methods:
  at home, 246–248
  in restaurants, 12
  stomach cancer and, 224
  in weight-control plan, 84–85
Copper, 155, 163–164, 170, 204, 255
Coronary bypass surgery, 53
Coronary heart disease (see Cardiovascular disease)
Coumarin as flavoring agent, 176
Crash diets, 63
Cream (see Dairy products)
Crude fiber, 200, 203
Cutback maneuvers in calorie-control menu, 78–80
Cyclamate, 173, 174, 177
Cystic fibrosis, vitamin E for, 156
Cytosine, 24

Dahl, Lewis K., 108, 109
Dairy products, 8
  in calorie-control menu, 77
  carbohydrate content of, 36
  cholesterol content of, 136, 138–139
  exchanges for, 82, 84
  in fad diets, 63
  in low-cholesterol, modified-fat diet, 141
  protein content of, 24–26
  in prudent diet, 238
  saturated fats in, 25, 26, 137, 138, 235
  shopping for, 244–245
  as snacks, 42
  in sodium-restricted diet, 117, 118, 122
  in vegetarian diet, 227
  vitamins and minerals in, 152, 164–168
  weight control and consumption of, 82, 238
  when eating out, 244
Dancing, 75
Death:
  from alcoholism, 209
  from cardiovascular disease, 132, 134
  from G6PD-deficiency anemia, 159
  hypertension and, 102–104
  obesity and, 52–54
  from vitamin A poisoning, 156

Dehydration in air travel, 16
  (See also Water)
DeLuise, Mario, 60
Depression:
  amphetamine withdrawal and, 66
  exercise for, 71
  and magnesium deficiency, 168
Dermatitis (see Allergies and dermatitis)
Desirable weight, chart of, 55–56
Desserts (see Sweets and desserts)
Dexatrim, 68
Dexter, James, 216
Diabetes, 5, 6, 45
  caffeine and, 215
  cardiovascular disease and, 137
  chromium deficiency and onset of, 170
  diet pills and, 68
  dietary fiber and, 9, 199
  obesity and, 47, 52, 54
  primary treatment for, 10–11
  sugar intake and, 39–41, 219, 236
  triglyceride levels and, 143
  underweight as symptom of, 94
  vitamin B_{15} for, 160
  vitamin C megadose and, 159
  vitamin E and, 156
Diarrhea:
  caffeinism syndrome and, 217
  due to mannitol, 177
  due to thyroid compounds, 67
  due to vitamin megadoses, 157
  and excessive fiber intake, 204
  potassium deficiency and, 168
  and sodium needs, 114
Diastolic pressure, 102
Diet (see specific types of diets)
Diet pills, 66–68, 91
Dietary cholesterol, 8, 9, 14, 32, 132–140
  in balanced diet, 235–236
  in calorie-control menu, 81
  in controlled-carbohydrate, modified-fat, moderately re-
    stricted cholesterol diet, 144
  in eggs, 32, 136, 138, 235
  healthy intake of, 135–138
  in low-calorie, low-cholesterol diet, 53
  in low-cholesterol, modified-fat diet, 140, 141
  in meats, 14, 32, 136, 139
  need to control intake of, 138–139
  new evidence on effects of, 133–134
  in prudent diet, 238–242, 257
Dietary fiber, 8, 9, 37–38, 193–205, 221, 222, 233–234
  in balanced diet, 236
  benefits of, 196–197
  carbohydrates as source of, 34, 200, 202
    (See also Carbohydrates)
  cardiovascular disease and deficiency in, 195, 196,
    198–199
  chemical composition of, 200
  colon cancer and, 38, 194, 195, 198, 221–222, 236

Grains and grain products (*Cont.*):
cholesterol content of, 136
decreased consumption of, 9
dietary fiber in, 194, 202–204
exchanges for, 82
in fad diets, 64
in home-prepared meals, 248
low-calorie, 79
in low-cholesterol, modified-fat diet, 141
in low-sodium diet, 115, 117, 118, 122
protein content of, 23–26
in prudent diet, 240
shopping for, 245
in vegetarian diet, 227, 228
vitamins and minerals in, 152, 155, 166, 168, 170, 171
weight control and consumption of, 82, 240
Greden, John, 217
Growth retardation, manganese and zinc deficiencies and, 171
G6PD (glucose-6-phosphate dehydrogenase) deficiency, anemia and, 159
Gums, vegetable, as food additives, 178, 180
Gums (oral cavity), bleeding, vitamin C dose reduction and, 158

Habit belly, obesity due to, 59–60
Hair loss, vitamin A megadose and, 156
Hangovers, caffeine for, 216
Hashim, Sami A., 91
Hayes, Arthur H., Jr., 16, 114
HDL (*see* High-density lipoproteins)
Headaches:
caffeine withdrawal and, 215
in caffeinism syndrome, 217
diet pills and, 66
MSG and, 177
vitamin megadoses and, 156, 157, 159
Health foods, 147, 148
natural foods as, 147, 188–190
prices of, 181–182
(*See also* Organic foods)
Health Promotion and Disease Prevention, Surgeon General's Report on, 71, 194
Healthy People (Surgeon General's Office), 208
Heart attacks, 32, 53, 219
alcohol and, 205–207
atherosclerosis and, 125
coffee and, 214
hypertension and, 99, 104, 237
incidence of, 99
obesity and, 19, 51
vitamin E in prevention of, 156
Heart muscle, effects of potassium deficiency on, 168
Heart rhythm disturbances, 65
alcohol and, 210
amphetamines and, 66
caffeine and, 215
due to thyroid compounds, 67

Heart rhythm disturbances (*Cont.*):
effects of potassium deficiency on, 168
low-carbohydrate diet and, 65
Hegsted, Mark, 7
Hemorrhoids, 38, 197
Hepatitis, alcoholic, 209
Herbert, Victor D., 187
Herbs and spices, 250–252
as low-calorie additions to weight-control plan, 84
in low-sodium diet, 115, 117, 118, 122, 123
Heredity (*see* Predisposition)
Hernia, hiatus, 38, 197
Heyden, Siegfried, 214
Hiatus hernia, 38, 197
High blood pressure (*see* Hypertension)
High-calorie foods for underweight problems, 95–96
High-density lipoproteins (HDL), 127–131, 172
effects of alcohol on, 207–208, 210
High-fiber diet, 202–204
High-protein diets, 63, 161–162
Hippocrates, 148
Histidine, 23
Hives (*see* Allergies and dermatitis)
Holoenzymes, 149
Home-prepared meals, balanced, 245–253
Hot baths for weight loss, 69
Humectants as food additives, 179
Hydrogen cyanide, 174
Hydrogenated fats, 32, 33
Hydrogenation, defined, 32
Hypercalcemia, 167
Hypertension (high blood pressure), 5, 6, 10, 99–124
alcohol and, 210
atherosclerosis and, 104, 105, 128
borderline, incidence of, 100
coffee and, 214
dietary fiber and, 9
due to nonprescription diet pills, 68
heart attacks and, 99, 104, 237
incidence of, 110, 237
kinds of, 105
mortality and, 102–104
overweight and, 18, 19, 51, 52, 59, 105–108, 116
salt intake and, 9, 105, 108–112, 219, 237
and need to reduce salt intake, 16, 111–112, 115–117
vitamin B_{15} for, 160
Hyperthyroidism, underweight and, 94
Hypertriglyceridemia, 142
Hypoglycemia, vitamin E megadose and, 160
Hypotension, air travel dehydration and, 16

Ideal diet (*see* Balanced and varied diet)
Ideal weight, 9, 57
Idiopathic (essential) hypertension, 105
Impotence, diet pills and, 66
Incidence:
of atherosclerosis, 125
of borderline hypertension, 100